D1686413

Roll This!

The Best Foam Roller & Acuball Guide You Will Ever Own

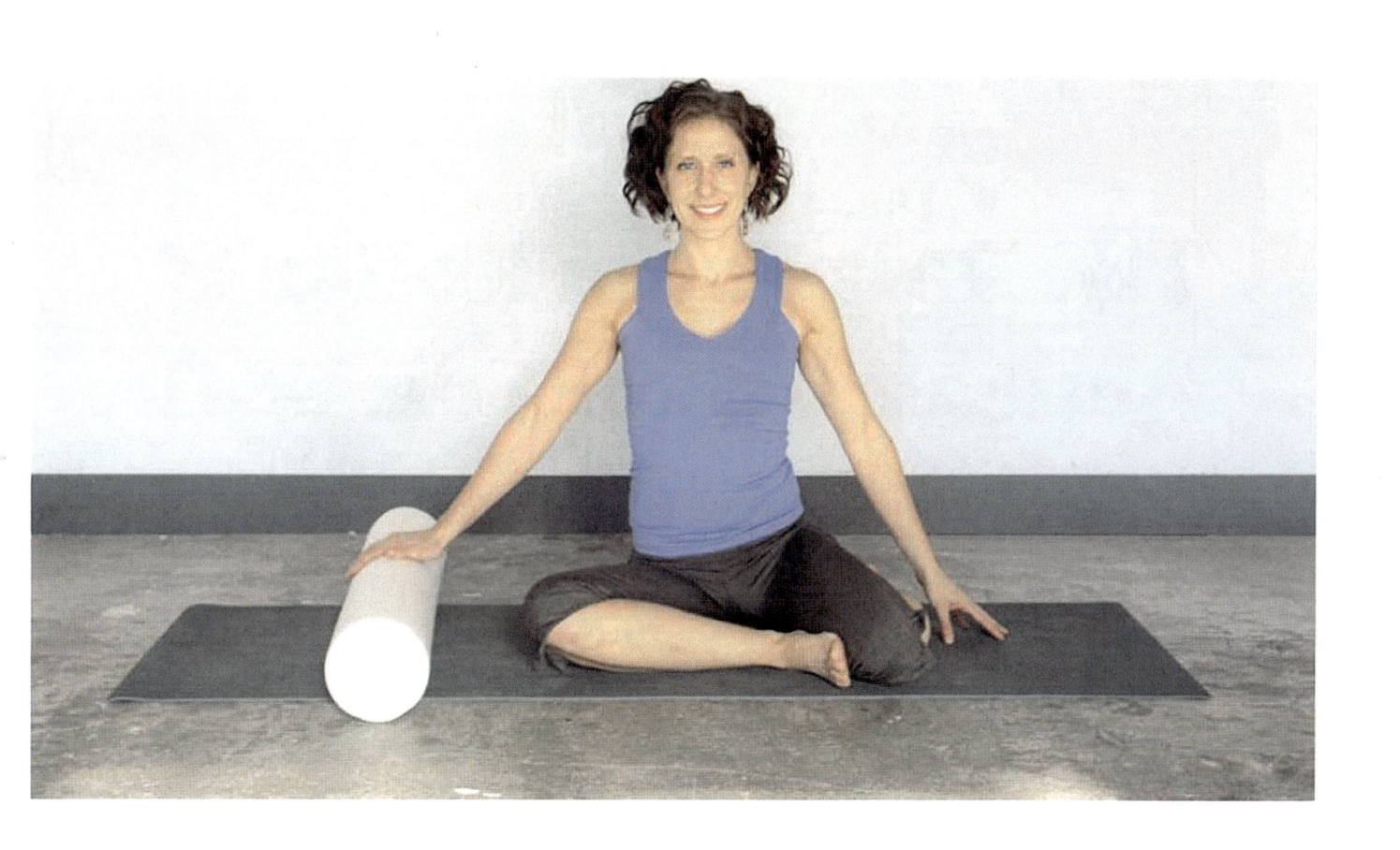

Roll This!

The Best Foam Roller & Acuball Guide You Will Ever Own

Hope Zvara

Author's Note: The book proposes a program of exercise recommendations for the reader to follow. However, you should consult a qualified medical professional before starting this or any other fitness program. As with any diet or exercise program, if at any time you experience any discomfort, stop immediately and consult your physician.

©2016 Copper Tree Yoga Studio & Wellness Center in works with
Hope Zvara & Core Functional Fitness by Hope Zvara® all rights reserved

Photography done by Chloë Gribbin-Scharpf and Artists Eyes Photography, Carol Grant-Stevens.

To book trainings or workshops with Hope for to schedule her for a full weekend training using this manual contact her below:
1364 E Sumner Street
Hartford, WI 53027
www.HopeZvara.com
www.HopeCoreFitness.com
info@hopezvara.com

In gratitude to my students,

without their everlasting support and encouragement-

that I have changed their lives,

I would not be able to give this gift to all of you.

Contents:

Pages:

11	Acknowledgements
14	Why *Roll This!*
15	Why the Foam Roller and Acuball
16	Breathing in your Foam Roller Practice
17	Rolling and Mayo Fascia
18	Stability VS. Mobility
19-21	Finding Neutral
22	Resting Position

Warm-Ups:

23	Pelvic Tilting
24	Spine Rocking
25-26	Neck Massage & Release
27	Occipital Release
28	Face and Chest Massage
29	Protraction-Retraction (Shoulder Blade Massage)
31-32	Foot Massage & Plantar Tendon Release

Spinal Release Series:

33-34	Lower & Middle Back Massage
35	Low Back Release & Sacral Massage
36-37	Middle (Thoracic) Back Release
38	Scapulae Release

Mayo Fascia Release Techniques:

39	Triceps Massage
40	Forearm Massage
41	Palm Rolling and Hand Release
42-43	Latissimus Dorsi Massage
44	Devotional Release
45	Camel (Lower Back Release)
46	Gluteal Massage
47	Sacral and Sacroiliac Release
48	Figure Four (Hip Rotator Massage)
49	Adductor (Inner Thigh) Massage
50-51	Hip Flexor & Quadriceps Massage
52-53	Supine Psoas Release
54	Prone Psoas and Iliac Release
55	Groin Release in Bound Angle
56-57	IT Band and Outer Thigh Massage
58	Outer Calf & Shin Massage
59	Hamstrings Massage

Foam Roller Arm Series:

60	Arm Scissors & Arm Extension
61-62	Arm Circles

63	Deltoid Fly
64-65	Pectoral and Biceps Curl
66-67	Triceps Extension
68-69	Weighted Triceps Extension with Heel Drop
70-71	Weighted Triceps Extension with Core Flexion

Supine Stabilization Series:

72	Basic Leg Extension
73-74	Single Leg Stretch
75	Single Leg and Arm Stretch
76	Core Supine Marching
77-78	Articulating Spinal Bridge
79	Shoulder Bridge
80-81	Shoulder Bridge Variations
82-83	Leg Circles
84-85	Foot Push
86	Leg Scissors
87	Heel Touch

Plank Series:

88-89	Stretching Cat (Swimming)
90	Plank
91-92	Knee Pull: Double
93-94	Knee Pull: Single
95-96	Pike
97-98	Push-Up
99-100	Reverse Plank

Forearm Plank Series:

101	Forearm Plank
102	Forearm Push & Pull
103	Forearm Plank Hip Twist

Side Series:

104	Side Plank
105-106	Side Kicks: Up and Down
107	Side Kicks: Front and Back
108-109	Side Kicks: Circles
110	Side Kicks: Bottom to Top
111-112	Oblique Lift
113-114	Mermaid Side Bend
115	Side Push-Up

Extras:

116-117	Rolling Lunges
118	Boat
120	References and Resources
121	About the Author

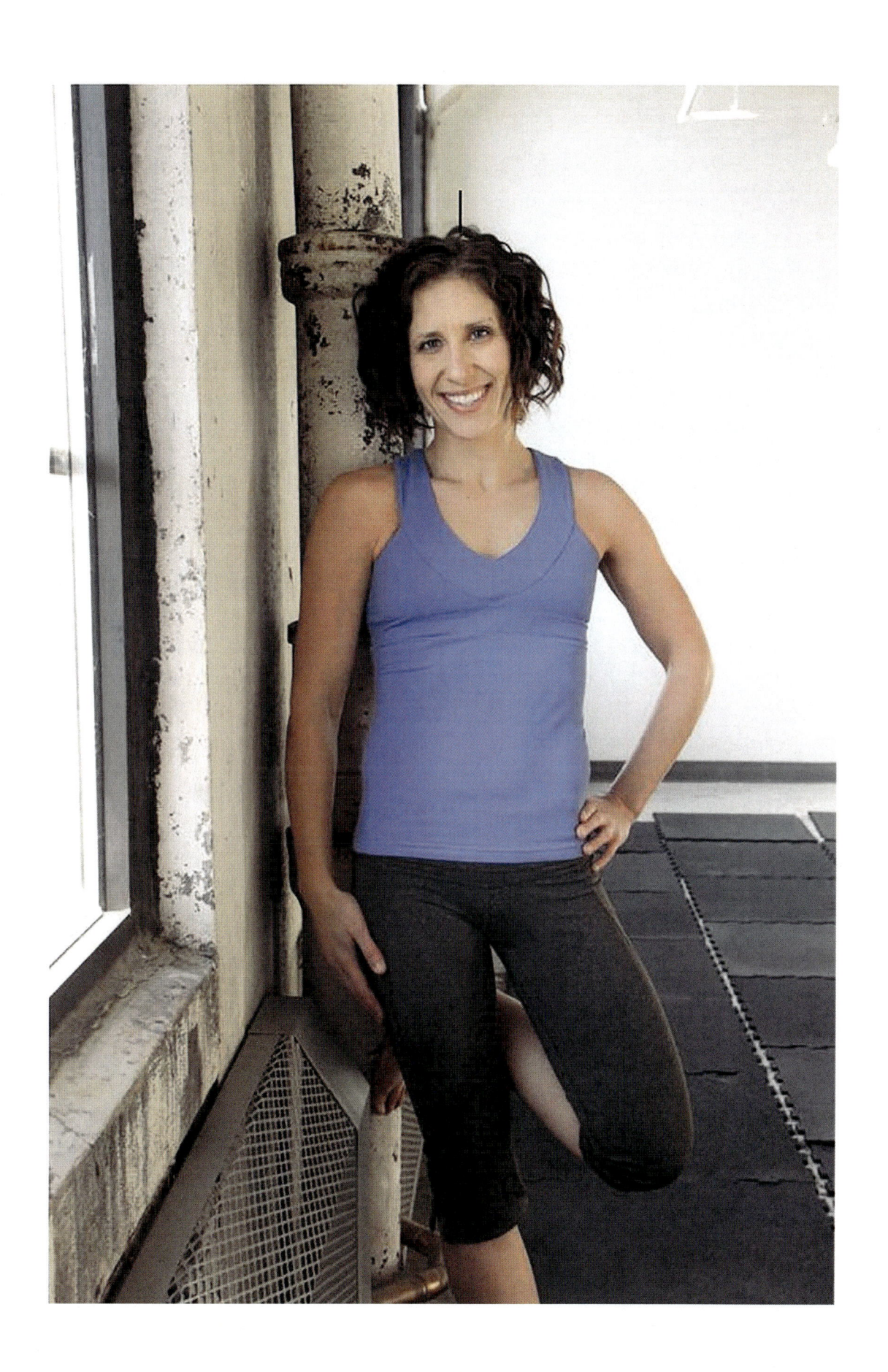

Acknowledgements:

The writings of this book would not have been possible without the initial spark given by my greatest influential yoga teacher, Swami Omkari Devanada. At the age of 19 she was placed in my life at a time I needed what she had to offer more than any other time. And my time with her over the following several years had not only changed my career path, but changed me as a person. She was truly the spark that taught me how important it is to teach yoga as a life practice and to not be afraid to allow yoga to spark spirituality in people. And although this book is not based solely on yoga, I would not have written this manual if it wasn't for her.

    I would also like to recognize my students and their trust and belief in me as their teacher and mentor. Over the past decade I have been told by many, *"I have a gift and that I am unlike anyone they have ever met, an old soul in a young woman's body",* and I am humbled and excited that the gift many tell me about I am now able to share it with people across the globe.

    I would also like to acknowledge my photographer, Chloë Gribbin-Scharpf; my husband's most talented cousin, who out of the goodness of her heart shot these photos in efforts to help me share my insights and passion for what I do, and Carol Grant-Stevens whom which has shot many, many photographs of me doing what I love.

    Finally, I am most grateful for the most supportive family any person could ask for. My husband, Brian, whom has supported me, my dream and business since the beginning; my three beautiful children, Harper, Meredith, and Ivan that without them and the drive to show them hard work, effort and how important it is to follow your heart and dreams, none of this would be possible.

12

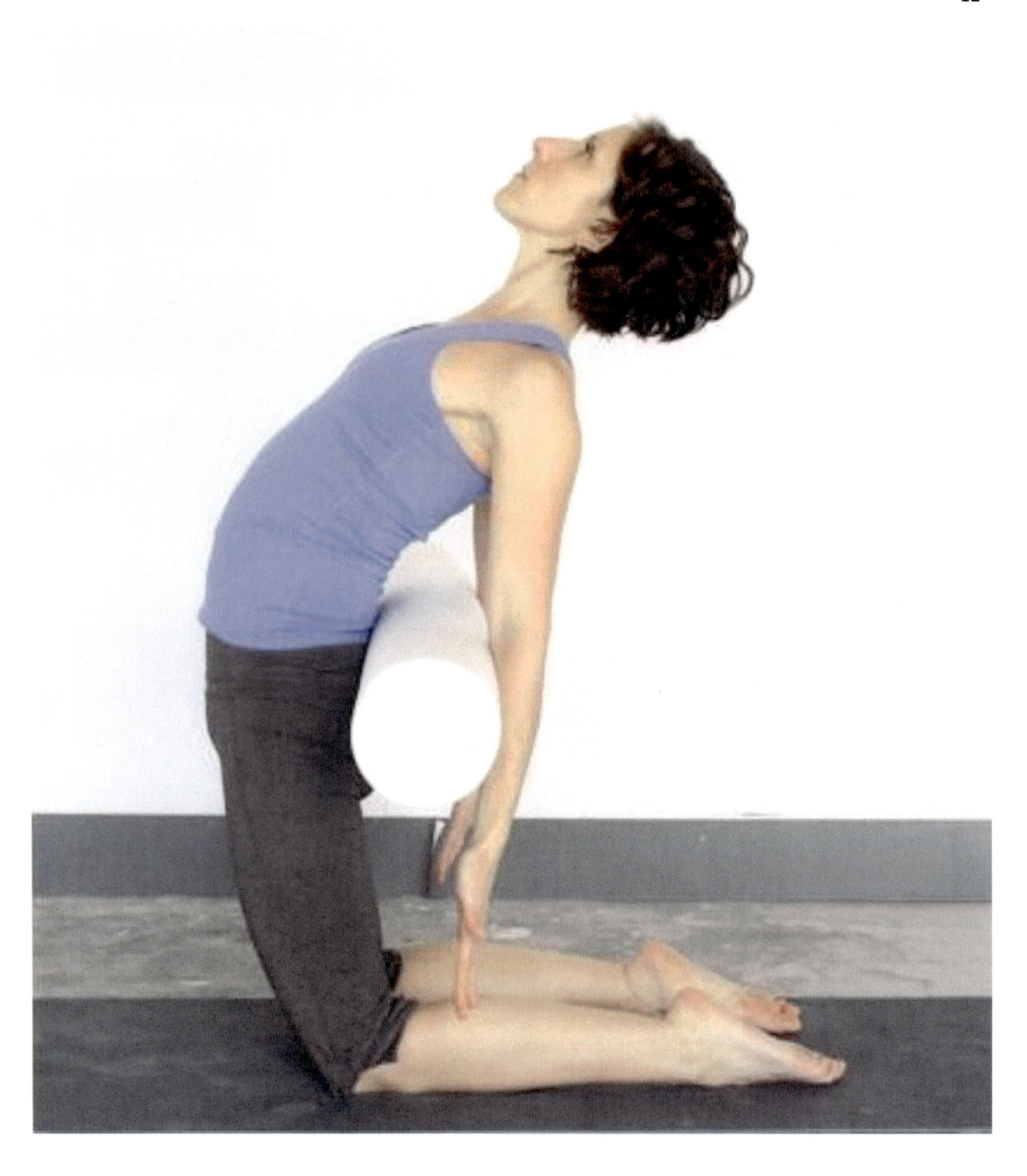

Why Roll This?

In my experience in the yoga and fitness world over the past decade, I have come to realize one of many things. As a yoga teacher, few teachers themselves feel confident and educated enough to incorporate props and different exercises into their teaching, allowing their students more variety and tools to then go home and apply.

Secondly, those teachers do not have enough information and training on the topics they are trying to teach, and thirdly, the students thirsty for this knowledge feel the lack of direction both from the teacher and from sources like books, videos, and workshops. They are given the bare bones basics, which is good, but only for a while. As a yoga teacher, movement enthusiast and the creator of Core Functional Fitness®, I see this need and frustrated myself, I decided to create a step by step easy to follow workbook for the foam roller and the acuball®. This workbook will allow all who use it the ability to feel confident about these tools both in a classroom setting and at home.

As a teacher, I recognize that our students are in fact our greatest teachers. Through their teachings and my listening, I am able to guide them into movements and exercises that actually help them instead of hurt them. And in truly listening to what they have to say as people and what their bodies say in class, I feel it is vital for me to share with everyone my findings and how my method of communication has now changed the lives of so many of my students as well as my own.

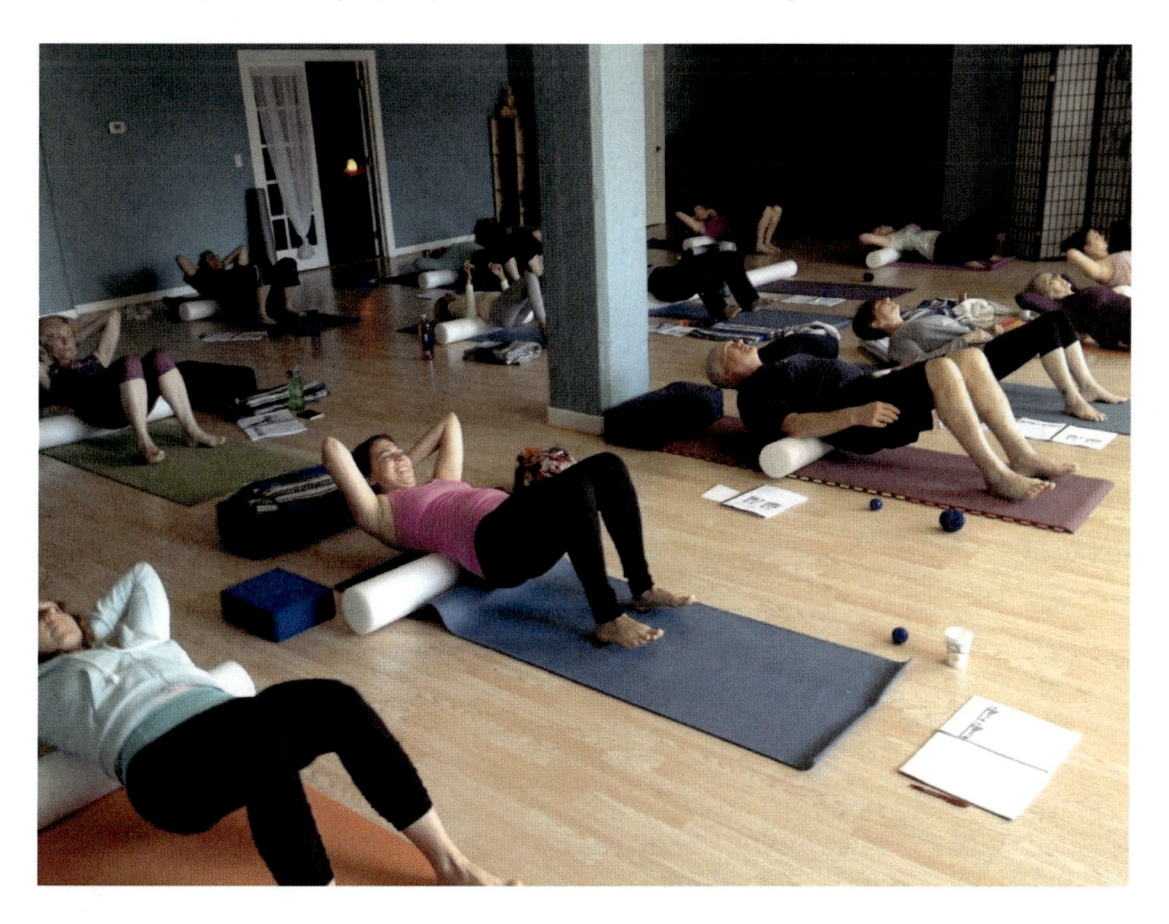

Why the Foam Roller and acuBall:

Today's fitness world is jam packed with foam rollers. Short ones, long ones, thick ones, thin ones, rollers with texture, and rollers so hard they could crack a tooth. Here, I am simply suggesting a standard (brands and places to purchase are at the back of this manual) foam roller. Some call this the softest foam roller, and that may be so, however, if your body is already bound tightly, you will not need something as hard as a rock. Many may notice bruising, high levels of discomfort and even pain when using a roller and that quite frankly may be too firm. As a teacher, you always want to acknowledge your most basic student and not only are the softer rollers cheaper, but they are the most user-friendly. When selecting a roller, please use your digression. Even when using a standard/soft roller, your tissues will still be happy and adhesions worked out.

Dr. Cohen's acuBall is a patented design that features 100% natural acupressure and (optional) heat. When using the acuball you are able to stimulate the acupressure points that then send a signal to the central nervous system, allowing one to benefit on an even deeper emotional level. The acuBall created by Dr. Cohen is a great partner to a foam roller, but a staple for all my classes I teach if someone is working to "stretch" an area but that area is stuck, coupling with rolling makes stretches, poses and movements more achievable and doable.

In using a foam roller and Dr. Cohen's acuBall, you can unlock areas of the body in ways such as:
- *Loosening tight muscles and joints*
- *Increased blood flow*
- *Improved digestion and elimination*
- *Calming to the central nervous system*
- *Removal of blocked energy in the body and deep set trauma*
- *Allows the brain to give and receive "feel good" signals to help one relax*
- *Renewing your proprioceptors that send signals back to your brain*

Using the foam roller for strengthening and core-based work allows you to enhance your performance in ways such as:
- *Working on a non-stable surface which allows us to access our deepest core stabilizers*
- *Teaching you stability before mobility to encourage proper core firing patterns, balance and stability.*

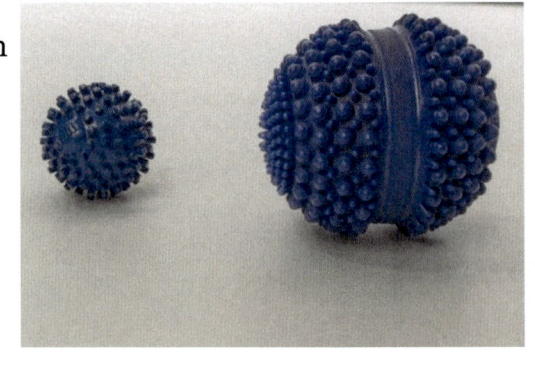

> *Offers a deeper awareness of the misuse of muscles in mat work.*
> *Offers increased feedback to understanding neutral during exercises, which allows increased body awareness.*

Breathing In Your Foam Roller Practice:

Breathing is an important element in any successful practice, physical exercise or not, the most important thing to remember *is to keep breathing.* Depending on how you will be adapting the foam roller into your practice may predetermine how you choose to breathe. Either in and out through the nose (more yoga based) or in through the nose and out through the mouth (more cardio or Pilates based).

In the massage-based techniques described in the book, nose breathing may be more appropriate as it is much more relaxing and releasing and as you see fit, exhaling out the mouth to help with areas of tension. In the strength or core building exercises, nose and mouth breathing may be more appropriate to accentuate the core contraction. This is not a manual on breathing, so all in all, please follow the breath cues and overall - just keep breathing. Our breathing cues are merely suggestions to help students guide themselves through the movements with ease.

Please note that new research is now showing that an important feature of co-contracting the abdominal muscles is the ability to do so independently of any lung ventilation patterns; and that in doing so we are training ourselves to breathe freely while maintaining abdominal bracing of an isometric stabilization contraction (McGill, 1957).

Understanding Our Fascial System:

- Myofascial pronounced *my-o-FASH-e-ul* is muscle + o + fascial, many will use the terms interchangeably but most are meaning the same thing: fascial system, myofascial, fascia to most mean the same thing.

- Myofascia is the combination of muscle and fascia, smoothing this relationship of tissues is an important point to be aware of in that releasing of such in the body can increase range of motion, flexibility, mobility and decrease pain.

- The practice of rolling is a fascial release technique that is meant to break up tight fascia in the body. Fascia covers our entire body much like shrink wrap surrounding our muscles, blood vessels, and nerves. Fascia is a type of connective tissue that wraps around the muscles. Everything was once connective tissue a combination of collagen and elastin.

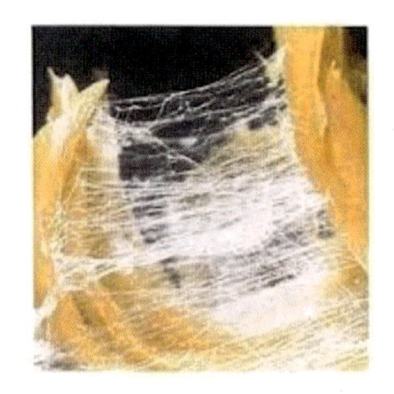

- Another way to consider our body is bags, in bags in bags. This concept holds to the idea that our muscles and bones are held in place by our fascial system, and when you readjust the bags, the muscles and bones go back to where they belong - what you learn in this workbook can help with just that.

- Is fascia dead? Well some say yes, and some say no. Fascia is excreted by living cells, much like a spider spitting out webs, it is very central to many processes in the body. Nevertheless, fascia is vital to everything; fascia has embedded sensory preceptors that correlate back with the brain for a full body response.

- Most injuries are fascial injuries, as fascia encompasses our body on numerous levels.

- When fascia is dehydrated, it will feel bumpy or sticky like, in that your muscles don't move well. Techniques like rolling can help with that.

- It is important to understand that foam rolling does not change the length of tissue, but rather it helps release the tissue from being stuck to unstuck.

- It is also important to note that adding more pressure, or texture to a practice of rolling and working with the fascial layer will not increase the results, but rather look at the sensory response to the technique used, start soft and see if you can feel in response to that action first. Most people need more pressure and texture to feel the action, this is in part because our sensory preceptors are deadened, try to feel more by doing less.

- Techniques like rolling with an acuBall or foam roller is a wonderful way to help break up scar tissue, soft tissue adhesions and trigger points that someone like a massage therapists would work on. Rolling is a wonderful technique to implement prior to a massage or chiropractic adjustment to allow the therapists to get more work done in less time and help the adjustment stay.

- When you use a foam roller or acuBall you are allowing the connective tissues to rehydrate, the nervous system to rebalance, the inner organs to detoxify, and our largest organ to be nourished - our skin.

- When using the foam roller or acuBall please be aware that working on one area of the body for more than ten minutes is not ideal. It's too much for the tissue in both mayo fascia release and when practicing other such exercises. *(Example: lying on your back using the foam roller for various exercises).* When rolling, consider a ten-minute warm up for the muscles and a ten-minute cool down to help prevent soreness.

- Many of us in today's society are dehydrated leaving our bodies very "sticky" underneath our skin (think two pieces of shrink wrap rubbed together). So, by working mayo fascia and then the combination of plenty of water, our bodies can begin to resume the balance they are meant to have. A good recommendation of daily water intake would .6 x your body weight in ounces. *(Example: .6 x 150 = 90 ounces, and if you are active it would be more).* In addition, adequate protein and Vitamin C are both important for a healthy fascial system.

Stability, Mobility and Core Work:

- When working through the sections in the manual on strength, stability and core work, it is very important to maintain neutral, and only work to a level that is comfortable yet challenging to you personally during that session of practice. Remember, we are all working the same muscles just from a different place. It is not healthy to over work the body in any way. You should always consult a physician when starting any new exercise routine. If possible, use this manual in coordination with a certified and experienced teacher to help you find variations that are most suitable for you.

When reviewing the exercises in this manual, it is important to understand that the purpose of these exercises is not to be thought of as *performed*, but rather seen as retraining exercises, movements, techniques and intelligent training for the body, mind and breath; through these practices developing balanced strength, core awareness and release in your entire body's tissues.

- The goal of this section of the manual is to help assist students in the *differentiation process*. This process is that we are aware of both the body parts that are moving and the body parts that are not moving. Many move as one unit, and although everything in our body is connected it does have an amazing ability to move separately. Through the process of differentiation, we then cultivate body awareness. Real body awareness is that in which one can think and feel during a movement and assist the body in activating, feeling, or releasing a muscle, joint or emotion that is currently the focus of the exercise.

- ***2:1 Ratio***. This is an important concept when working to create balance in the body. Doing simply equal on each side will always leave one side stronger. The 2:1 ratio asks that after practicing on each side that you go back to the weaker side and work through the exercise again on that side.

Finding Neutral:

- Lying on your back with the foam roller underneath the entire body from head to tail align the body so that all six curves (remember if the spine curves one way it has to curve back the other way) of the spine are aligned and neutral pelvis and neutral spine are achieved.

- Align your feet so that they are hip-width apart. This is simply the width of the bones beneath the fleshy gluts. You can easily find these by taking your fingertips to the lower gluteus of the body and pressing to find the boney landmarks. This narrow stance will challenge balance and our core stabilizers

- Bring the hands to the anterior (front) pelvic triangle of the body. Fingertips to pubis bone and heels of the hands to the ASIS (anterior superior iliac spine). This will setup your lumbar (low back) in neutral. This will leave you with a bit of space between your lumbar and the foam roller anywhere between the sizes of a grape to a golf ball. We all have differently spaced vertebra and different size torsos so this will be different for everyone, however, the process to align is the same for all.

- Relax the front of the rib cage down with a generous exhale to align the bottom of the ribs with the ASIS, which will set up your thoracic (mid-back) in neutral).

- Adjust the head and neck so that the eye line is angled up and slightly towards the body, not away and overhead.

- Allow the arms to fall alongside the foam roller. There are three main arm alignment options and these can be used interchangeably throughout your practice.

    - Palms and forearms down flat. This is the most supportive.
    - Palms down and forearm and elbow lifted with the eye of the elbow (this is the soft fold of the elbow) facing gently upward.
    - Palms facing inward towards the foam roller with the pinky edge of the hand on the floor and forearm and elbow hovering fully lengthened. This is the most challenging option as it really challenges balance and stability.
    - Simply lying on the foam roller helps to realign the entire spine and torso. In many of HOPE Yoga and CFF™ (Core Functional Fitness by Hope Zvara®) it is coined as a "chiropractor in a roller", as it helps to realign any misalignments in the body, particularly the spine.

Ideally the entire body should be resting in alignment from the feet to the crown of the head. And as a rule of thumb you assess the entire body from the feet to the crown (from the ground up).

As you work through this manual please refer to this neutral section on how to find neutral whenever it is mentioned.

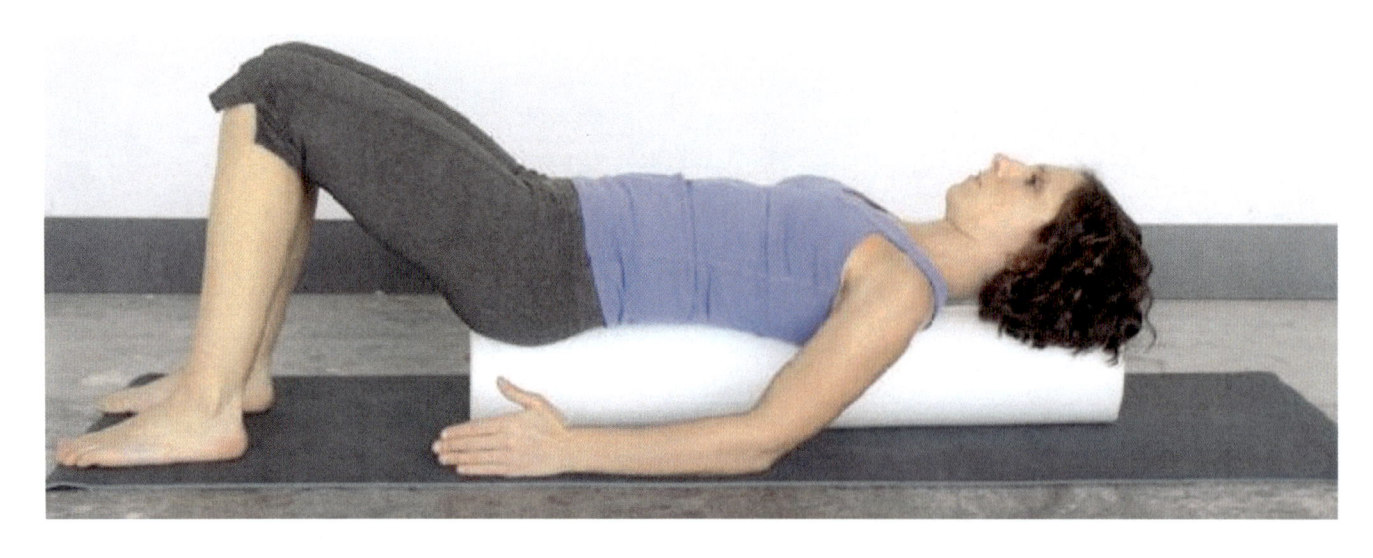

Neutral Alignment in Arm Variation 1

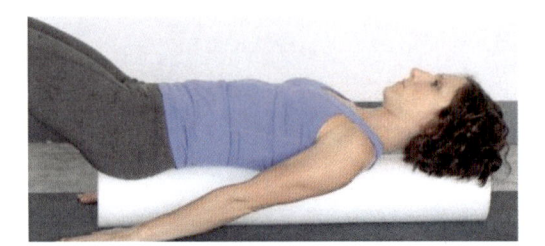

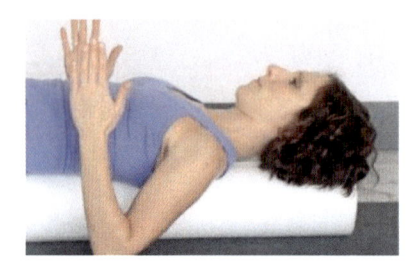

Arm Variation 2   Arm Variation 3   Arm Variation 4

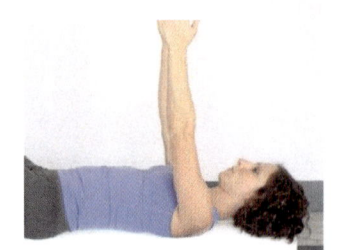

Lying supine (on your back) flat on the floor, palms up and limbs comfortably open away from each other. Take a few moments now and observe the body.

- How do you feel?
- Start scanning from the feet to the crown of the head.
- How does the body compare, right side to left side?
- Back side to front side?
- Does one hip feel higher or more restricted than the other?
- Shoulders elevated or depressed?
- Neck and chin level or is the chin pushed up towards the ceiling?

If you have a partner, ask them to now observe you lying on the floor. What do they notice? Feet, legs, knees, hips, ribs, shoulders, arms, hands, neck, head.

This simple basic awareness's will assist you in finding greater success in your foam roller practice.

Resting Position:
Resting on the foam roller from tail to crown, arms at your sides in an appropriate option that is stable, observe your body in a resting state. Review the previous observation points as discussed and now scan and observe your body on the floor. What is the current experience?

- What touches the floor and what doesn't?
- Where is there held tension?
- Where is there discomfort?
- Where is there a sense of ease?

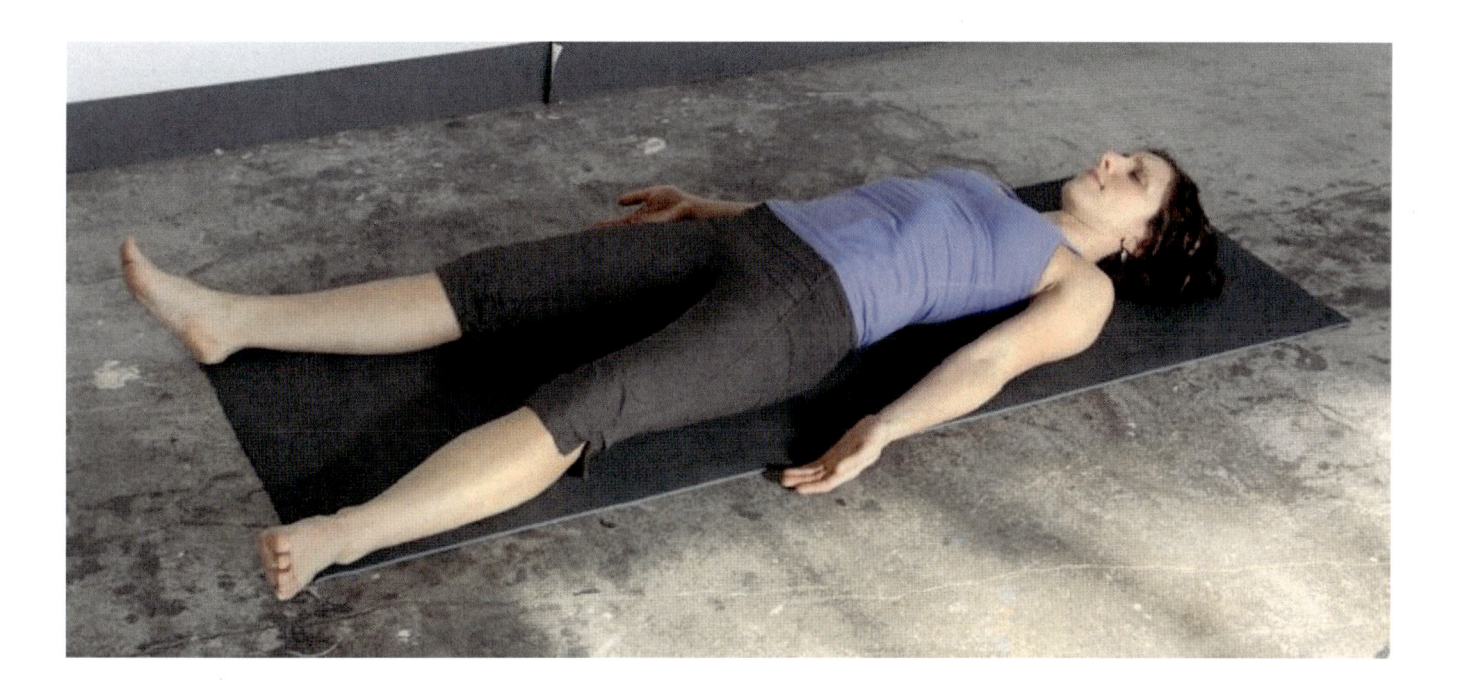

Pelvic Tilting:

To Begin:
- ➢ Lying on the foam roller align the body in neutral.
- ➢ Using the appropriate arm option find stability.
- ➢ INHALE and mindfully arch the lower lumbar (back) away from the foam roller, keeping the hips on the foam roller at all times.
- ➢ EXHALE press the lower back into the foam roller, feeling the pelvic-core (pelvic floor + deep core muscles) activate inward and upward massaging the inner belly and without squeezing the glutes.
- ➢ Repeat this series 10 times or up to one minute.
    - o *Variations:*
        - *Also, try this lying on the floor flat with your arms at your sides and your knees comfortably bent.*
        - *Try this when you inhale extend your arms over your head.*

Benefit:
This simple pelvic tilt is a great release on the lower back muscles and also on the SI joint (sacroiliac joint) which can be located running vertical, slightly above along each side of the tail-bone where the left and right iliac meet the sacrum. Here the spine connects to the pelvis. Pelvis tilts are one of the simplest things and more beneficial to do for lower back pain.

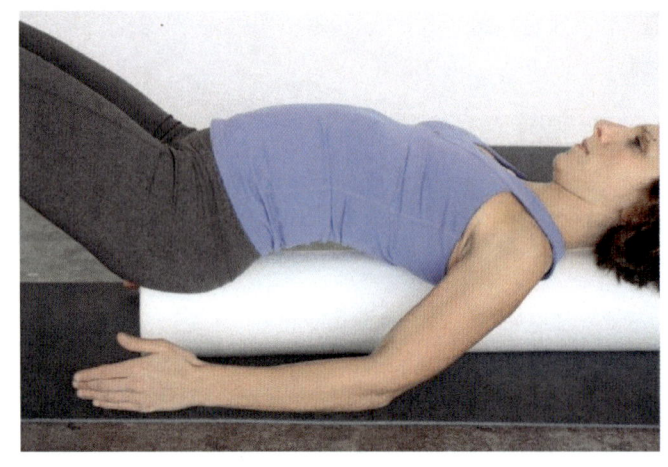

Pictured above: *Anterior Pelvic Tilt*. The body and low back are arching away from the roller.

Pictured at the right: *Posterior Pelvic Tilt*. The body and lower back are pressing into the foam roller, abdomen active.

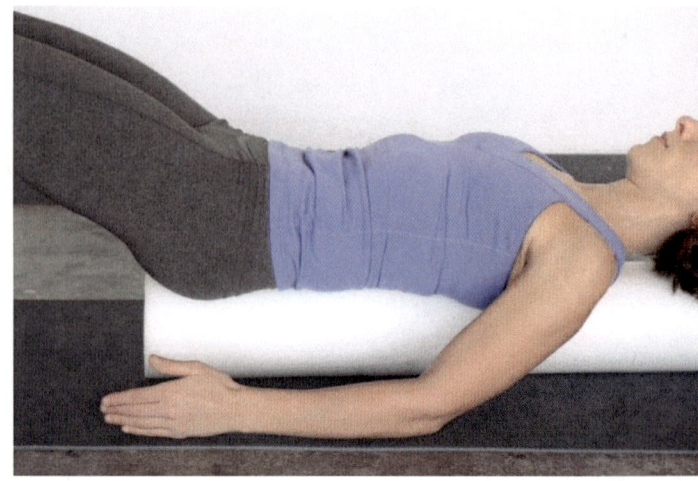

Spine Rocking:

To Begin:
- Lying on the foam roller align the body crown to tail on the roller in neutral.
- Only move in a way that feels right for your body in its current state.
- Keeping a regular breathing pattern, consciously begin to rock the body from the right to the left, massaging the muscles that surround the spine.
- Work to keep the core engaged not to fall off the roller.
- Notice how you feel and how the body reacts.
- If there is a point of tenderness or sensitivity pause on that point and keep pressure (trigger point) until it is released, continue to breathe, focusing on the exhale assisting the release.
- Continue this pattern for 30 seconds to two minutes.

Benefit:
    This movement helps to release all the muscles that surround the spine which and attribute to spinal misalignment along with shoulder and hip issues.

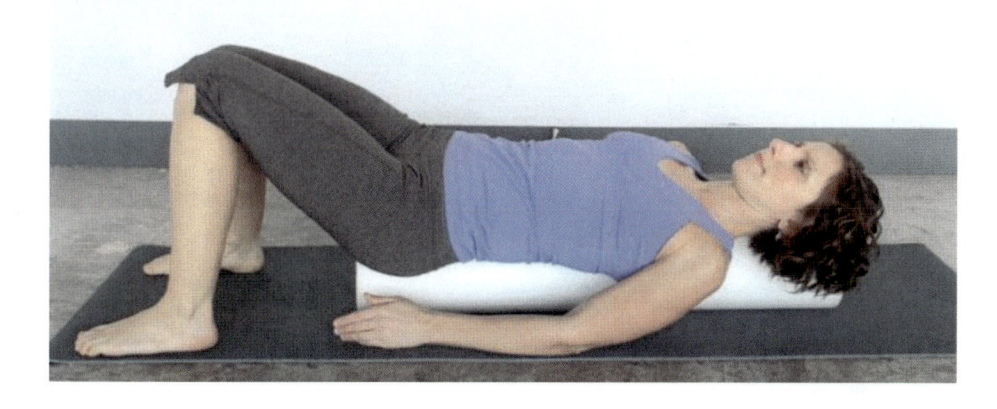

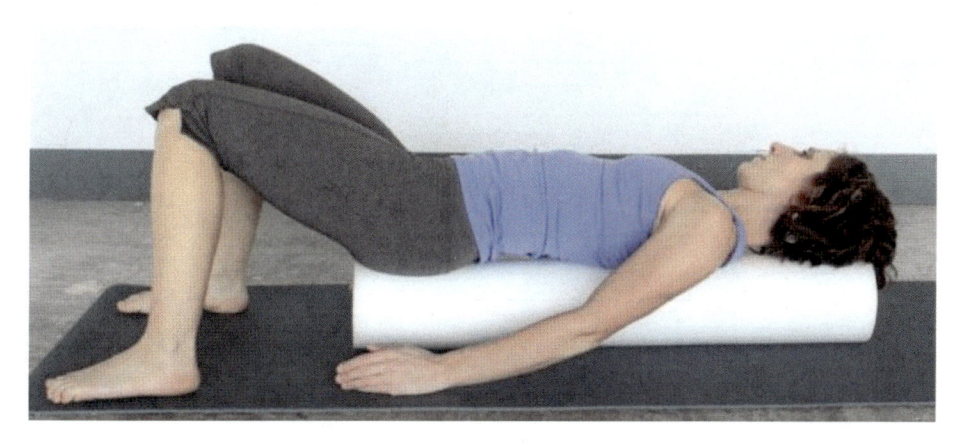

Neck Massage & Release:

To Begin resting flat on your mat:
- Lying in neutral on you back, find a comfortable arm position.
- Gently move the head right and left working to keep the shoulders relaxed.
- Notice how the head moves and if there is any restriction.
- Is it easier to move the head in one direction more or less than the other?
- Repeat this movement 5 to 10 times.

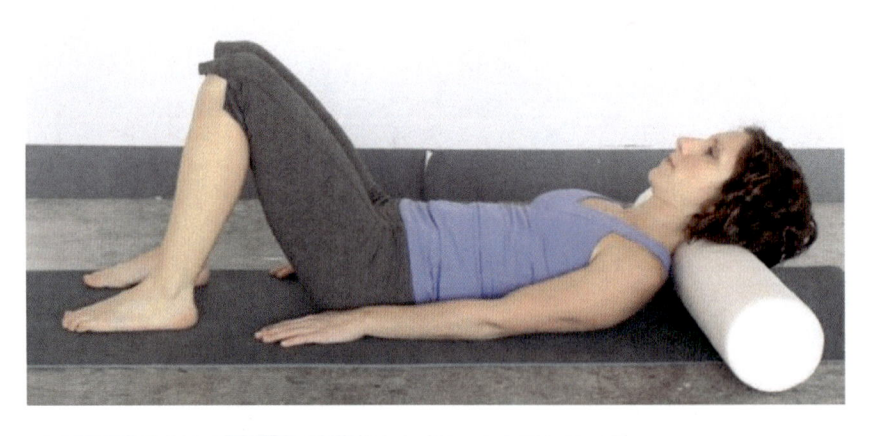

To Begin using the foam roller:
- With the foam roller running perpendicular with the body (like the cross of a "T") place the foam roller under the neck.
- Allow the rest of the body to rest on the floor in a supine position (on the back).
- Breathing comfortably; and begin to turn the head to the left and right.
- Pausing on any tender spots.
- Repeat this exercise for up to one minute.
  - *Do not perform if you have any major neck issues.*

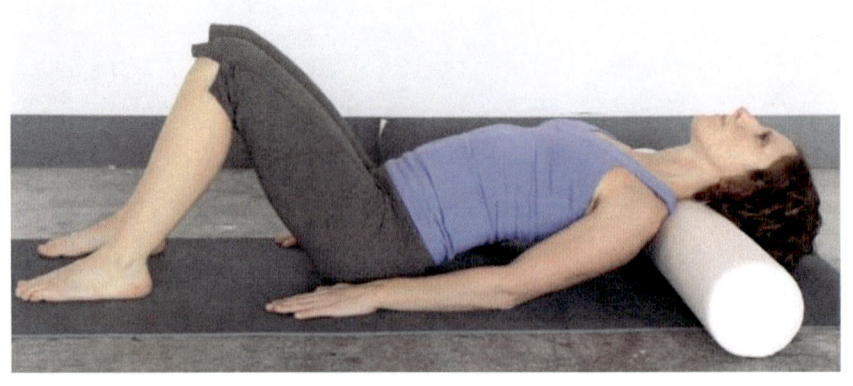

To Begin using the acuBall:
- With the large acuBall underneath the neck with the spine belt in line with your neck.
- Allow the rest of the body to rest on the floor in a supine position (on the back) with the knees bent.
- Breathing comfortably; begin gently roll on the acuBall allowing the cervical spine and attachments to release.
- Pausing on any tender spots.
- Continue this exercise for up to one minute.
  - *Do not perform if you have any major neck issues.*

Benefit:
- Here the muscles of the neck are released and the natural curve of the neck is emphasized.
- Those with shoulder and neck pain and those that clench the jaw or grind teeth will see a benefit in this simple, yet effective release.
- This is a great practice to consider for those with forward head issues or those who work a lot with electronics.

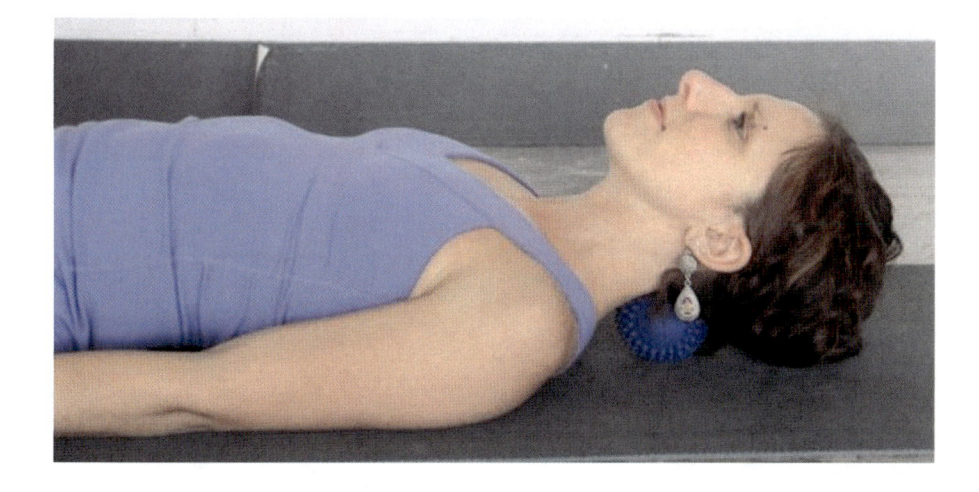

Occipital Attachment Release:

To Begin:
- Lie on your back with the body relaxing into the floor.
- Using one hand lift the head and place the acuBall underneath the bottom edge of the skull, the occipital bone.
- Adjust the ball so that the balls pressure points massage into the attachments of the muscles running up the back into the neck and base of the skull.
- When the ball is placed properly the chin will nod into the chest.
- Notice any knots by gently tilting the head to the right or the left or up and down.
- Once you find an area of concern pressure and hold, exhaling deeply or gently massage that area until the knot has released. Or gently rock the skull on the acuBall slowly to release any trigger points.
- Remain here for several breaths to several minutes until you feel the neck has released.

Benefits:
- The muscles of the trapezius and erectors of the spine feed into the base of the skull; this offers a great release into the neck.
- Those with sore necks may benefit with regular practice.
- TMJ, teeth grinders or those that clench the jaw may benefit from this release technique.
- Acts as a release for the levator scapulae at the attachment of the occipital bone.

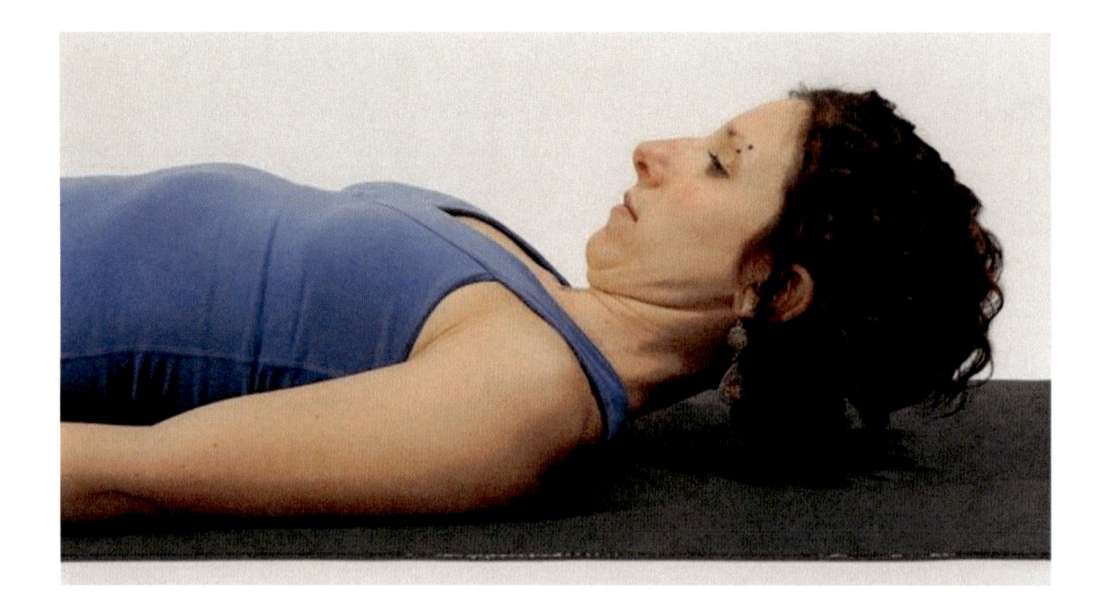

Face and Chest Massage:

To Begin:
- Lying down (or seated) take the small acuBall and begin to roll the ball onto the facial muscles.
- Start at the temple points on the outside of the corners of the eyes and continue to roll into the hair line as the temporal lobe extends beyond the corner of the eye.
- Continue rolling over the eyebrows into the third eye point (the center of the brows) over to the opposite temple point and up to the forehead and hair line.
- Roll down toward the jaw line and explore the joint of the mandible and maxilla, continue to move behind the ear and then down the jaw to the opposite side of the face.
- Roll the nasal pressure points on each side of the nose, adding pressure and holding as needed.
- Take a few more moments and explore the top of the head and any other area of interest.
- Set aside one to three minutes to work with facial massage.
- Then venture down to the chest and clavicle line roll the mini acuBall along the underside of the clavicle out towards the shoulder and over the chest for an additional one to three minutes.

Benefits:
- Facial massage with the acuball is a wonderful stress relief technique, great post workout (or pre-relaxation) and wonderful to help with stress relief before one goes to bed.
- Massaging the jaw line is extremely beneficial for those who suffer from TMJ and other like issues of the mouth and jaw.
- Stimulation to the muscles of the face and skull allows an increase in blood flow to the head and face.
- Facial massage may aid in a deeper more relaxed Savasana (Corpse pose in yoga).

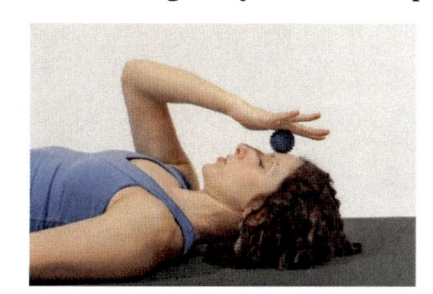

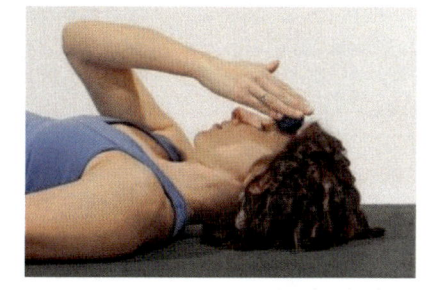

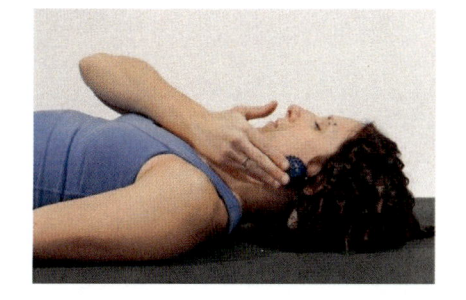

Protraction-Retraction (Upper Back Massage):

To Begin:
- Lie back on the foam roller and align the body from tail to crown.
- With the feet supportive in neutral, reach the arms over head vertical to the ceiling, palms face in.
- Without being on the elbows INHALE drop the shoulders around the foam roller, feeling them melt down.
- EXHALE with a strong core reach the finger tips up towards the ceiling feeling an exaggerated rounding in the upper back and shoulders.
- Continue to move in this method for up to a minute.
  - *Variations:*
    - *As the shoulders mold around the foam roller on the INHALE bend the elbows down to touch the floor.*
    - *Try this with the large acuBall in between the shoulder blades.*
    - *Try this in Bridge pose.*

Benefit:
- This offers a release of fascia from the upper back and spine particularly the space between the shoulder blades where the rhomboids are located.
- Muscles that support and restrict the shoulder blades are worked and released. This is a beneficial exercise to perform for anyone who is struggling with upper back kyphosis (a rounding of the upper back and shoulders, which is most of society in the west today).
- Winging in the scapulae, when the shoulder blades press out of the back rather than lie flat. Working with protraction retraction aids in reclaiming healthy upper back alignment.

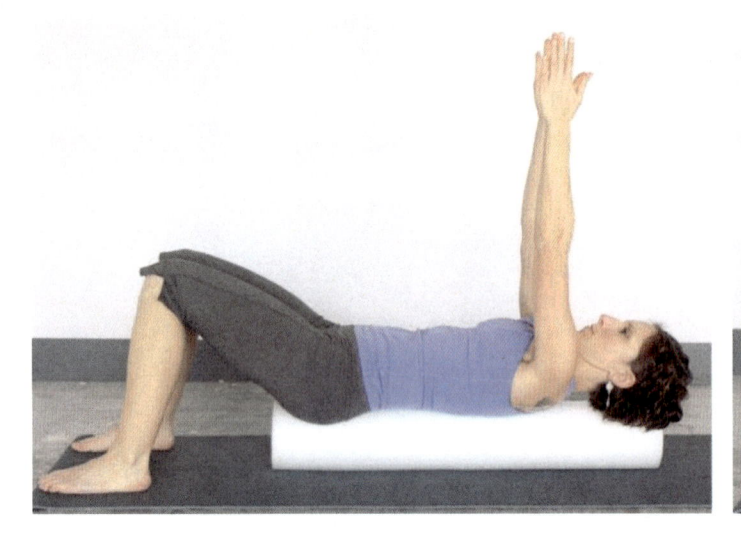

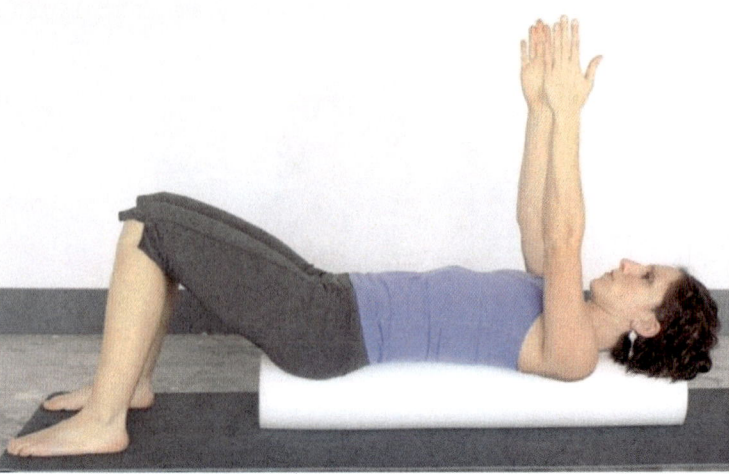

Protraction   Retraction

Front Chest Opening:

To Begin:
- Lying with the foam roller underneath you from crown to tail-bone align your body evenly on the roller and find neutral pelvis and spine.
- Find the feet at a comfortable hips width possibly with a support between the legs for better stability.
- Gently open the arms up to a cactus position, where the elbows line up with the shoulders and the palms are facing upward.
- Work to breathe deeply and relax the arms focusing on the shoulder and chest releasing and stretching.
- Work to remain here for one to five minutes.
- To release, gently draw your elbows to your sides and fold your arms over your belly.
- Gently roll off the roller to rest on your side.
    - *Variations:*
        - *If you have a tight front chest and the arms float, support the arms with rolled towels or blocks and slowly over time work your way down to a minimal support.*
        - *If this is too much try doing this flat on the floor with no roller.*

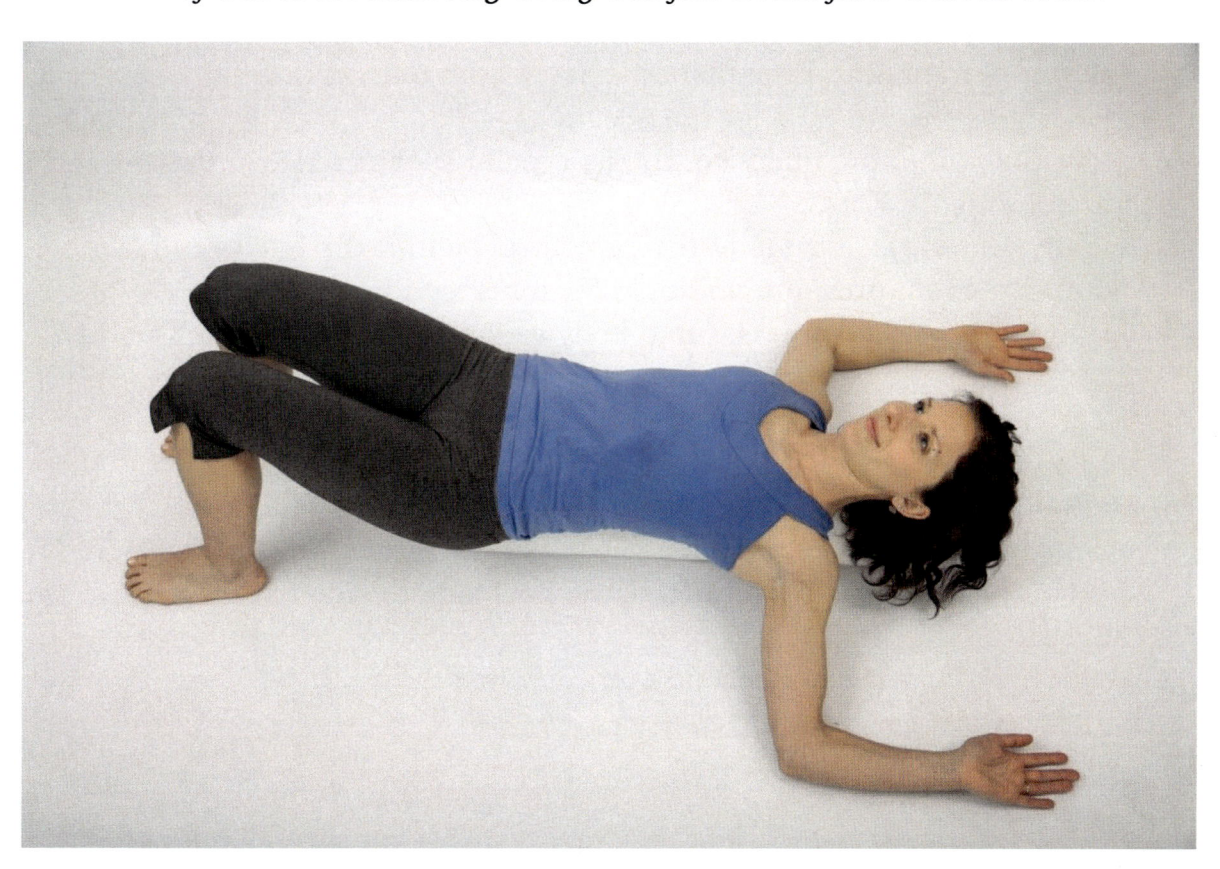

Foot Massage & Plantar Tendon Release:

To Begin:
- Begin standing with your small acuBall on the floor in front of you.
- Placing one foot onto the acuball™ begin to apply gentle pressure and roll on the ball.
- Breathing calmly, and explore all areas of the foot with the ball.
- Rolling on the heel, outer and inner edges of the foot, and ball of the foot.
- Noticing any areas of concern, pause and apply more pressure to trigger point the area allowing the tension to dissolve.
- Continue with this practice for 1 to 2 minutes.
- Then gently on an EXHALE fold from the hips into a forward bend notice how one hamstring has released simply by rolling the foot.
- Repeat the opposite side.
  - *Variations:*
    - *Try using the foam roller or the large acuBall.*
    - *Try balancing on the foam roller with both feet.*

Mini acuBall Plantar Tendon Release Technique:

- After rolling out the bottom of the foot for a minute or two, place the small ball in front of the heel on the plantar tendon (the tendon down the center of the foot), pressure and hold for ten seconds.
- Move the ball to the middle of the foot (solar plexus area), pressure and hold for ten seconds.
- Finally, move the acuBall to the point just behind the ball of the foot on the plantar tendon, pressure and hold for ten seconds.
- As your feet allow draw as much body weight onto the pressure point as you can manage and continue to breathe.
- Repeat the opposite side.

Mini acuBall Heel Grind
- Plant the ball of the foot into the floor and with the mini acuball™ under the heel of the foot roll the ball under the heel side to side to help release the hips and pelvis.
- Work here for ten to 30 seconds on each heel.

Benefits:
- It is important in any area of fitness and lifestyle that you work the feet. Many of us are in shoes all day (and shoes that don't fit), are standing or simply ignoring our feet.
- By rolling our feet, bound up fascia is released allowing the rest of our body to benefit.
- The 72 thousand nerve endings (nadis) on the bottom of the feet are linked up with organs and energy centers in the body, here, things like digestive concerns may be alleviated.
- Those with plantar fasciitis (a restriction of the plantar tendon), cramping feet, are standing, in shoes all day, or need a bit of a release; rolling on the feet is simple and the benefits travel to the entire body.
- Spending your day in shoes (with a positive heel) encourages the muscles and tissues in your feet to stop working as they should, this is meant to wake up those tissues.

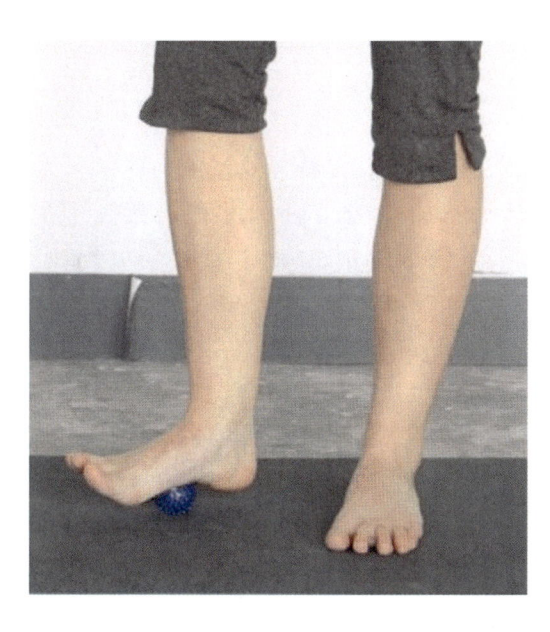

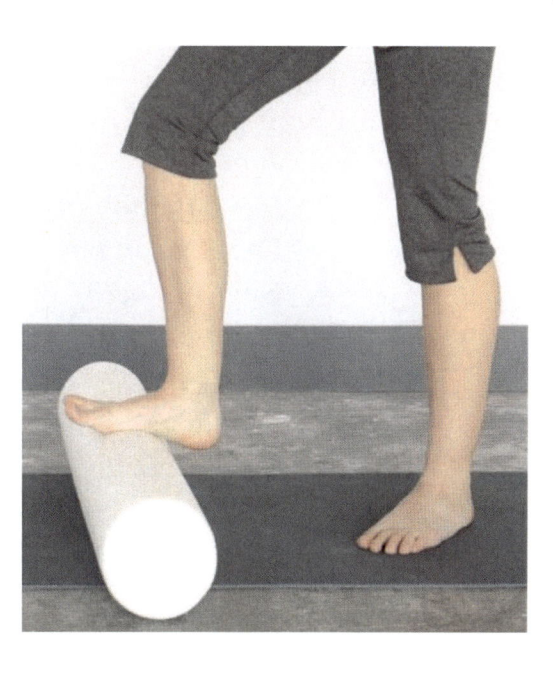

Spinal Release Series:
Lower & Middle Back Massage:

To Begin:
- Turn the roller perpendicular with the body and lie to the roller with your lower back on the middle of the foam roller and kindly hold the head in your hands.
- Breathing in and out calmly and regularly and begin to roll by pushing with the feet back and forth.
- First focusing on the lower lumbar and then working your way up the spine.
- Move slowly and when you come across a trigger point of tenderness or discomfort hold on that point and breathe deeply until the sensation fades.
- Experiment with rounding out the body to help hit all muscles of the back and spine.
- Continue with this rolling for one to two minutes.
  - *Variations:*
    - *Place the forearms on the floor behind the roller.*
    - *Focus in on one area of the spine and remain there.*
    - *Shift the body's weight to one side or solely focus on the left or right side of the spine more or less.*
    - *This can also be done with the large acuball on the floor.*
    - *Try this standing up against the wall with the foam roller or large acuBall behind the spine. Slowly bend and straighten the knees, leaning into the prop behind you.*

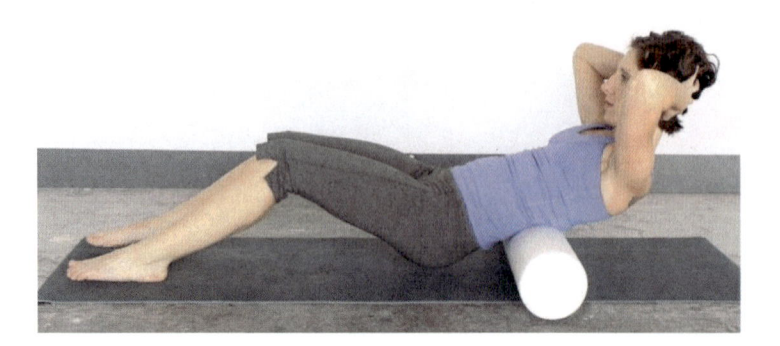

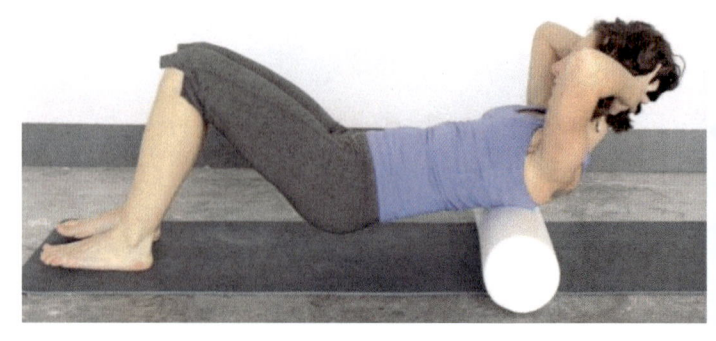

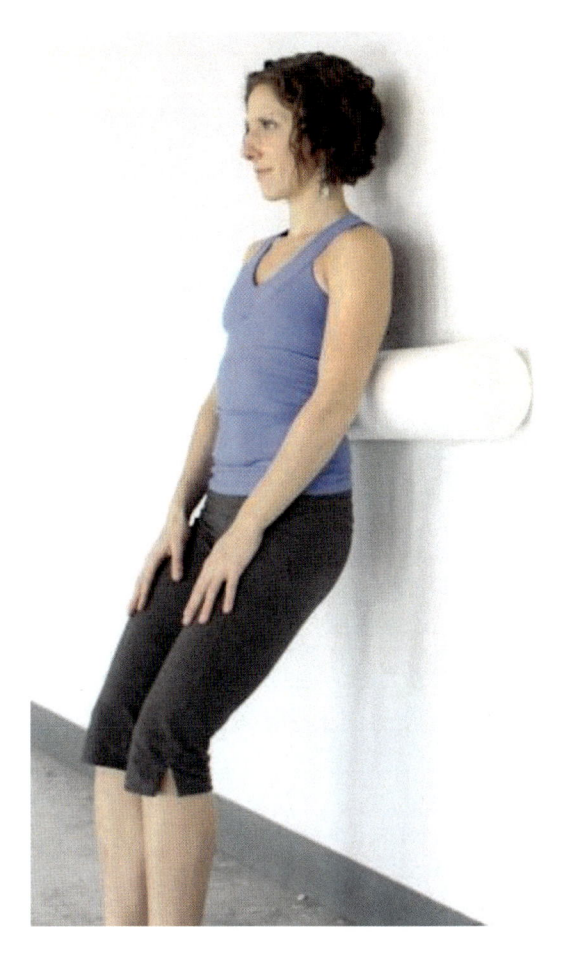

Rolling against the wall with the foam roller.

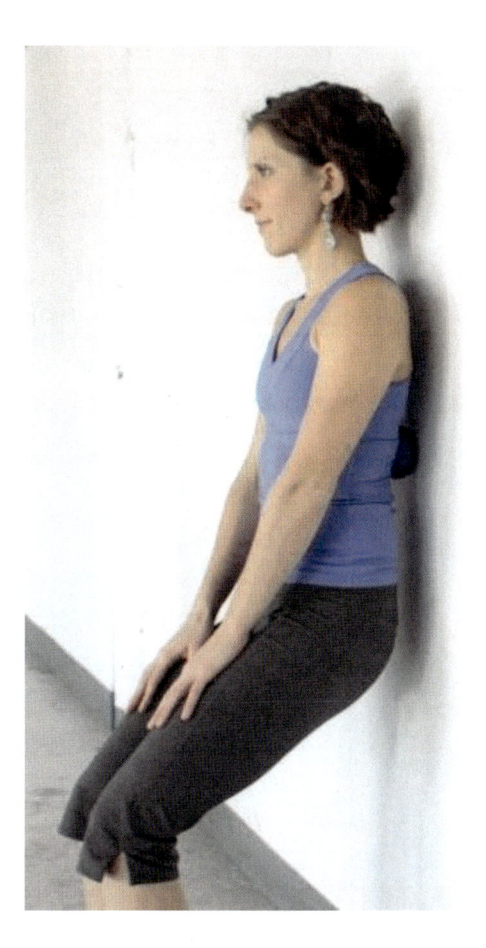

Rolling against the wall with the large acuBall or acuBack

Benefits:
- For many people, we live fairly sedentary lives with minimal movement, leaving our spines and muscles of the back stiff and tight.
- This movement can aid the erectors of the spine and rhomboids between the shoulder blades as well. This is a wonderful way to release those muscles and create more movement.
- The same is true for many athletes; too much emphasis is put on strengthening and not enough on release.
- This is a great exercise to do pre-massage and also pre-workout, to help release any restriction and fascia.
- Using the large acuBall and aligning the spinal rung in line with the spine, one may be able to realign twisted vertebrae and release tight erector muscles that run alongside the spine.
- Use either of these techniques pre-chiropractor and in between sessions to help your adjustments stick and last longer.

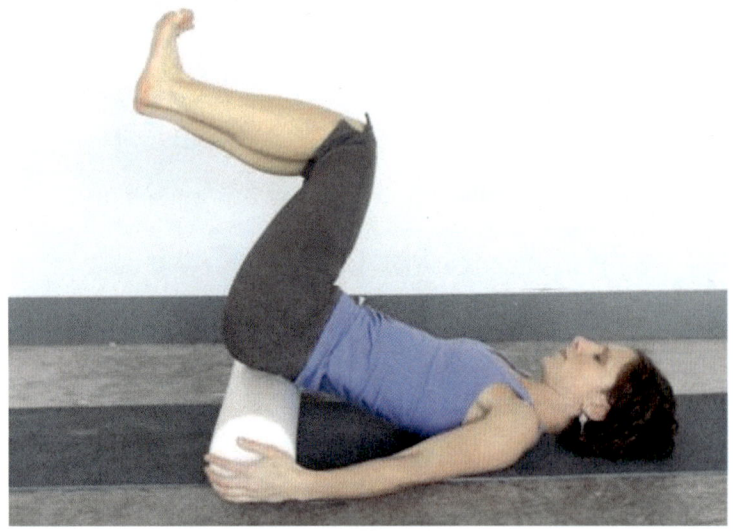

Spinal Release Series:
Lower Back Release & Sacral Massage:

To Begin:
- ➢ Lie onto the back and lift the hips to slide the foam roller perpendicularly underneath the hips and sacrum.
- ➢ Rest the hips onto the center of the foam roller.
- ➢ INHALE; lift the legs up and in towards the chest.
- ➢ EXHALE; allow the small of the back to round towards the floor, noticing a shift of the sacrum away from the lower lumbar.
- ➢ Hold here for a few breaths to help release the lower back.
    - o *Variation:*
        - *Gently rock the hips side to side.*
        - *Realign the knees above the hips as they rest on the foam roller. Gently rock side to side massaging the sacrum.*

Benefits:
- o The muscles of the lower back and sacrum are gently released and massaged.
- o This is great for those with lower back pain, SI joint instability, and women with menstrual back pain.
- o A gentle release of the muscles of the lower back.
- o Gentle core toning.

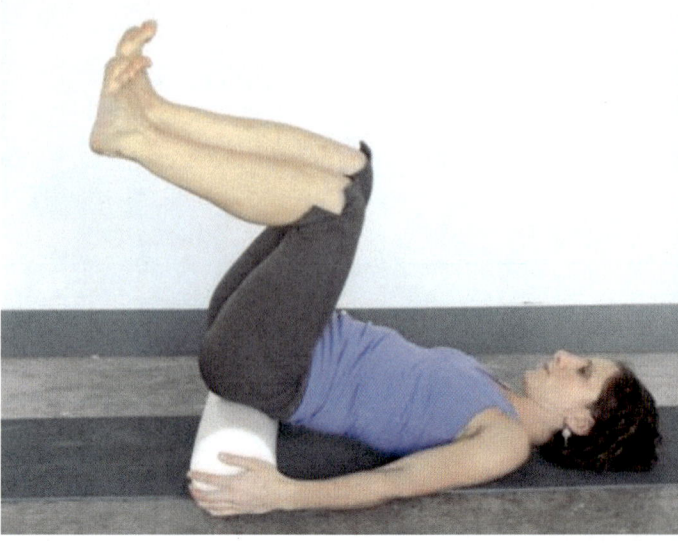

Spinal Release Series:
Middle (Thoracic) Back Release:

To Begin:
- Start sitting on the floor and place the foam roller crosswise behind you.
- Slowly lay back to where the foam roller hits the mid spine.
- INHALE; slowly begin to lie back supporting the head in the hands.
- If you chose to fully extend the arms parallel alongside the ears, however, do not force the arms to touch the floor or rest symmetrical, allow the body to release as it needs to.
- Completely release the torso over the roller allowing the rib cage to open and the breath to expand completely.
- If necessary place something under the head for more support so the neck does not strain.
- Use the breath to help release tension.
- Remain here for a few breaths up to several minutes.
- To come out roll to one side and press up.
    - *Variations:*
        - *Try this with a large acuBall or a mini acuBall.*
        - *Try the arms at "T" position or cactus for a different release.*
        - *Add a head support to aid in a gradual arching, especially if the upper back and shoulders are tight.*

Benefits:
- Here the front body is opened as much of our day to day postures are front body rounding.
- The rib cage expands and the muscles between each muscle called the intercostals muscles are stretched.
- This can be beneficial during pregnancy as the space beneath the rib cage can start to be compromised.
- Opening the chest and heart in this fashion can be emotionally challenging, it is normal in chest openers to feel emotional welling, remember to breathe and stay calm, do not stuff down any emotion that surfaces.

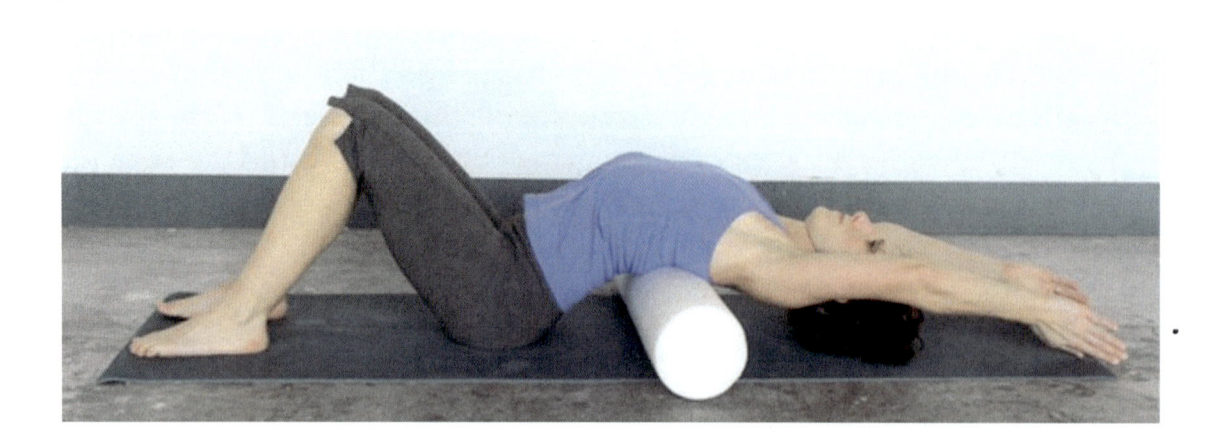

Release with foam roller

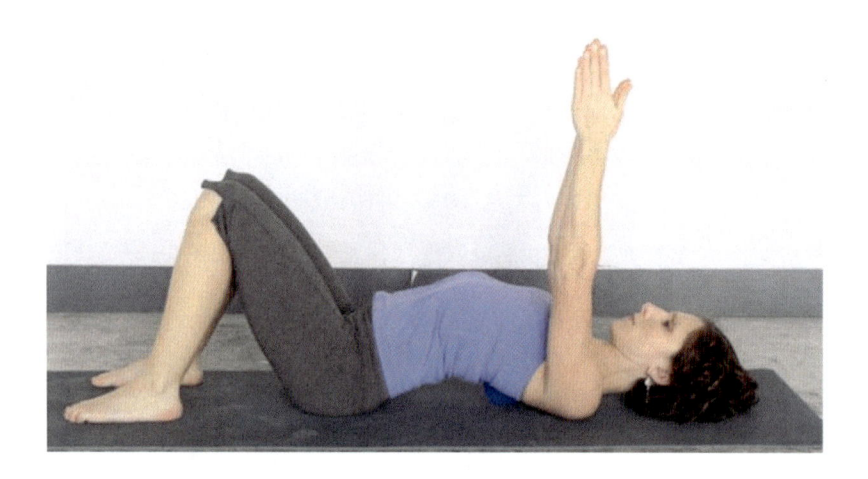

Release with large acuBall or acuBack

Scapulae Release:

To Begin:
- ➢ Lie onto your back and place the mini acuBall under the upper back lining the scapula (shoulder blade).
- ➢ Using your hips and feet to help move the body on top of the ball work to trace the shoulder blade looking for any tenderness, knots or restrictive areas.
- ➢ Reposition the acuBall as needed, upper scapulae, the column between the inner shoulder blade and spine, lower edge and outer edge.
- ➢ Repeat the release on the opposite side, treating each side as its own.
    - o Variations:
        - ▪ Try using the large acuBall placed along the spine lining up the spinal belt with the spine incorporate a pelvic tilt method to move the ball a few inches at a time.

Benefits:
- Releasing the scapula is necessary for proper shoulder joint movement.
- Often times shoulder pain and issue can be directly related to a scapula restriction, causing a referred pain (pain in an area that is not the area of injury or restriction). By working to release the shoulder blade you are allowing your body the opportunity to give freedom to the neck, shoulder and upper spine.

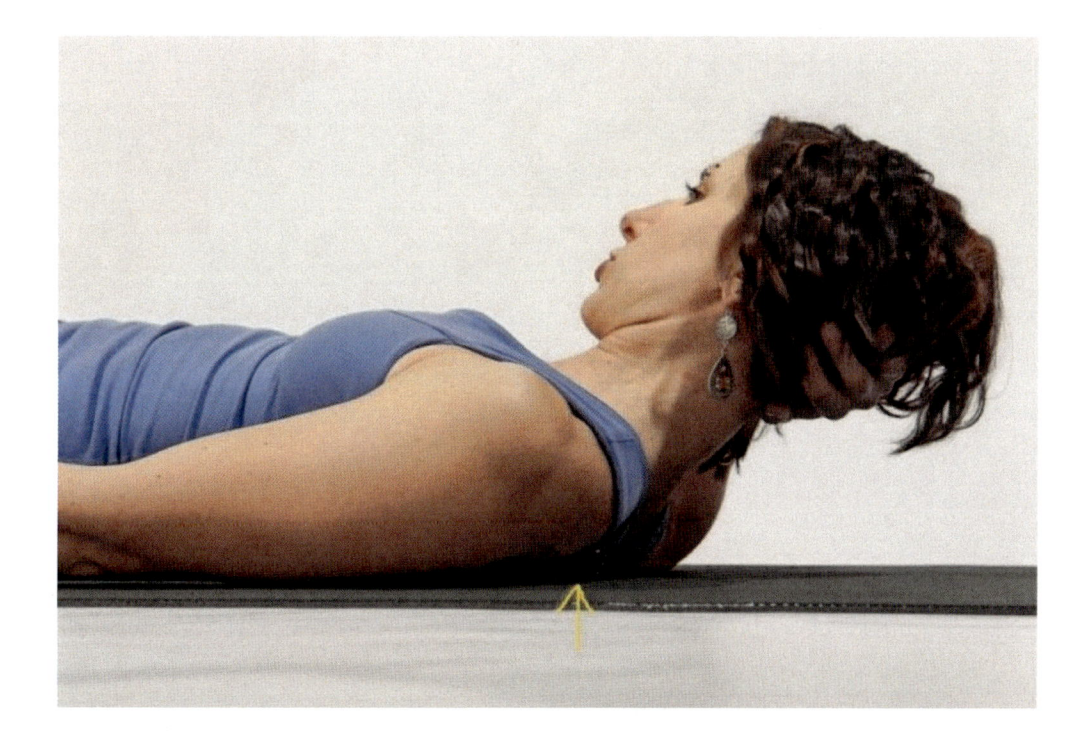

Triceps Massage:

To Begin:
- Lie onto your right side and place the foam roller crosswise above you.
- Place the right triceps (which is the back of the arm) onto the middle of the roller.
- Using the support of the left arm and hand in front of the body, gently begin to move your body back and forth feeling the upper arm gently massaged.
- Keep the core engaged for spinal support and position the head to reduce neck strain.
- Continue with this movement for up to one minute.
- Repeat on the other side.
  - *Variations:*
    - *Try this with the small or large acuBall.*
    - *If necessary, hold the head with the top arm for more support.*

Benefits:
- Here, the triceps are released and massaged helping to release the restriction of triceps into the shoulder socket.

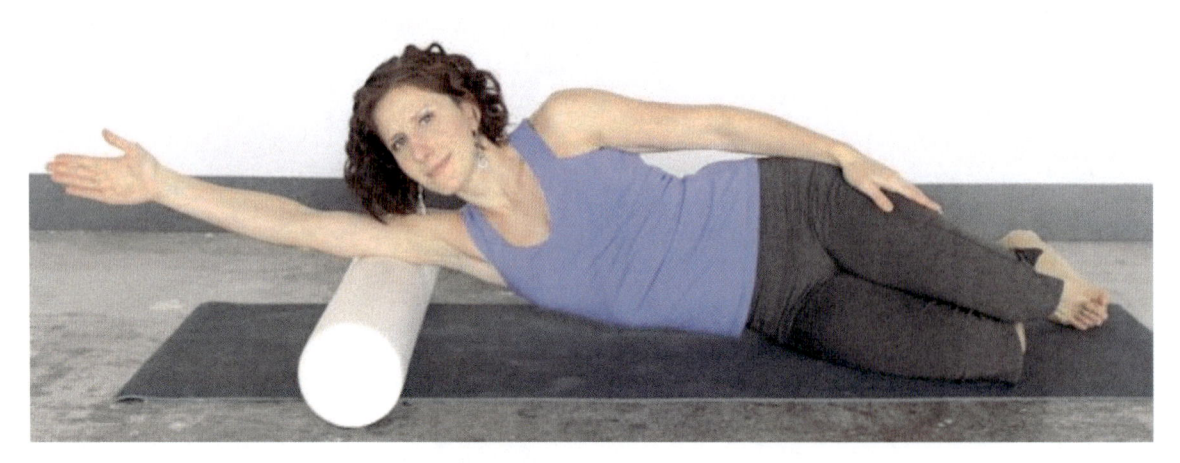

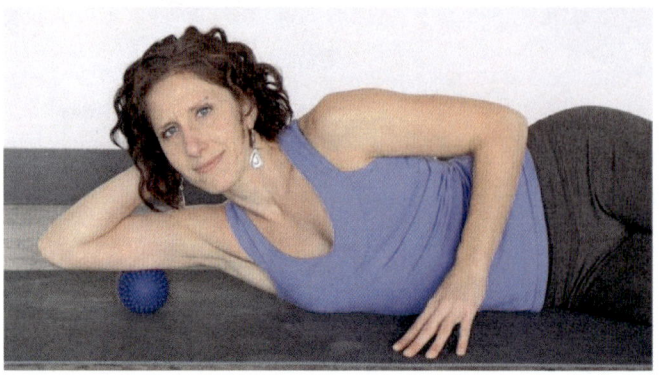

Forearm Massage:

To Begin:
- Come to a kneeling position and place your large acuball underneath one (or both if you have two) of the forearm(s).
- Sit back towards the heels.
- Breathe slowly and deeply paying close attention to any and all sensation in the body.
- Make the movements with the acuBall as large or small as your body sees fit.
- Work to roll from your wrist to the elbow.
- Pause in tender areas and apply gentle pressure to release bound up muscles.
- Continue to perform this movement for up to a minute on one or both arms.
    - *Variations:*
        - *Try this sitting at a desk or in a table top position (on all fours).*
        - *Try different aspects of the forearm: top, side, bottom*
        - *Try this with a foam roller or the mini acuBall*
        - *Try working with an open fist or closed fist for a different release.*

Benefits:
- The forearms are released and tightness leading to wrist strain or tennis elbow is alleviated.
- Major forearm muscles that both help to extend and flex the hands and move the fingers and thumbs are massaged and relieved (great anti-texting release).
- The muscles that often get overused in today's world with such activities like typing, texting, knitting, holding a hammer, and major repetitive strain injuries are brought back to balance here.
- Here Carpal Tunnel Syndrome (inflammation of the carpal bones) and tennis elbow is also relieved from this movement (take note that releasing the shoulder with issues like the above is vital to long-term stability and balance.

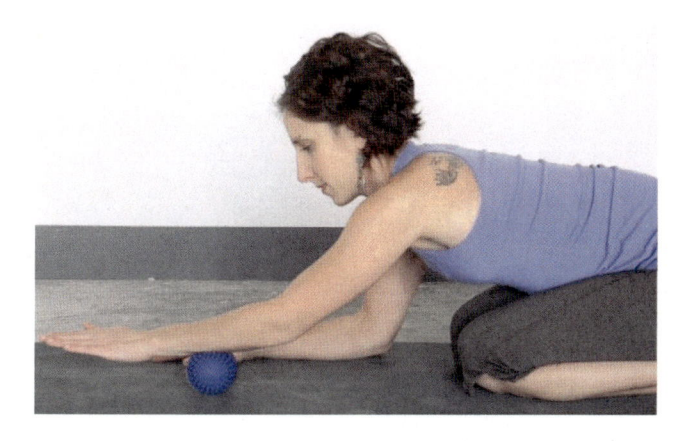

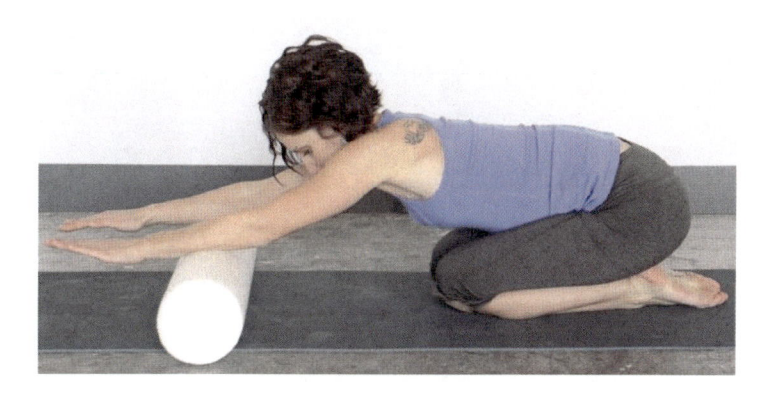

Palm Rolling and Hand Release:

To Begin:
- ➢ Place the small acuBall between the palms.
- ➢ Begin to roll the ball between the hands has hard or softly as your palms will allow.
- ➢ Work the entire palm, especially near the thumb and first finger.
- ➢ After a several breath of rolling the acuBall between the hands, cup the ball together in between the palms and press as hard as you can for five to ten counts.
- ➢ Release the acuBall and stretch the hands open.
  - o *Variations:*
    - *Do this with the ball on a flat surface and roll out the palm.*

Benefits:
- o The hands are over worked and carry a great deal of repetitive strain from things like computer work, texting, and various repetitive movements. Using an acuball regularly can help alleviate wrist strain, arthritis, and carpal tunnel issues where inflammation is present.

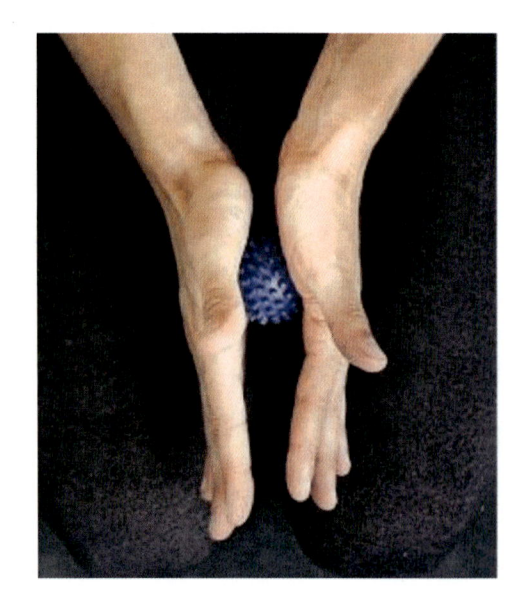

Latissimus Dorsi (Lat) and Teres Major and Minor Massage:

To Begin:
- Start by lying down onto your right side body, knees slightly bend up and place the acuBall or foam roller underneath your right arm pit.
- Kindly extend the right arm out running alongside your ear thumb facing upward.
- Gently roll out tracing the outer edge of the shoulder blade into the under arm cavity.
- Focus on tight or sensitive areas.
- Experiment with trigger pointing areas by just holding pressure to that point to calmly rolling the area out until sensation has decreased.
- Use the exhale to assist in the release of fascia (restriction in the body).
    - *Variations:*
        - *Try this against the wall*
        - *Venture to the lower scapula to find additional release*
    - *2:1 Ratio*
- Repeat the opposite side.

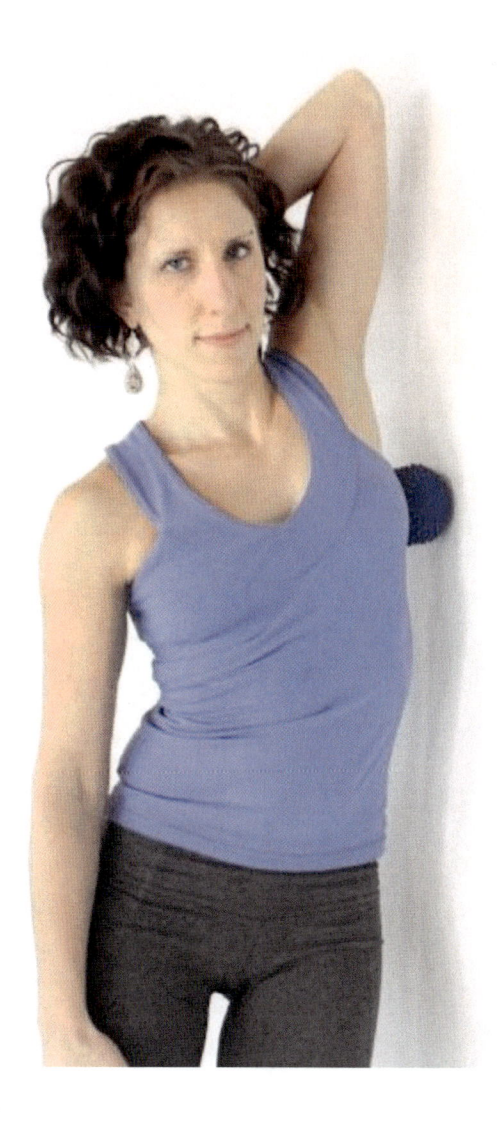

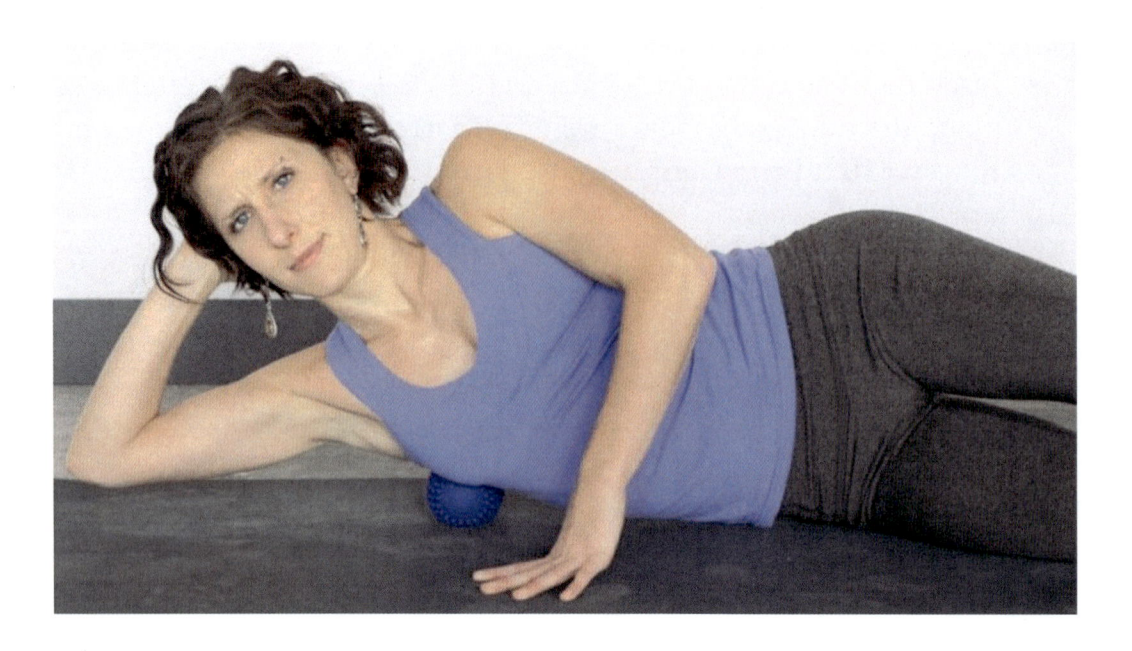

Benefits:
- Our latissimus dorsi connects from our lower body (iliac crest, sacral vertebrae, lumbar vertebrae and the last four thoracic vertebrae along with the three lower ribs and a portion of the scapula (also known as the shoulder blade). This very large muscle travels up the back of the body and comes under the arm to attach at the humerus bone (upper arm bone) on the bottom front side of the body. So simply put, when your lower back is tight or restricted this also puts a restriction on the opposite attachment site located at the humerus.
- Tracing the outer edge of the shoulder blade can also help to release teres major and minor two muscles that help keep the scapulae in place, but can often create restriction and tightness, limiting the shoulder blades range of motion and essential limiting the shoulder itself in range.
- Roll this area out daily to improve arm range of motion and all over comfort in the body.

Devotional (Lat) Release:

To Begin:
- ➢ Start in a table top position (all fours) with your hands on the foam roller.
- ➢ Exhale; sit back onto your heels as you move the foam roller out and away from your body.
- ➢ Continue to keep the core strong.
- ➢ Using your finger tips continue to roll the foam roller out to create a deeper stretch.
- ➢ Breathe gently and deeply, hold for up to one minute.
  - o *Variations:*
    - *Try shifting your hips off to one side.*
    - *Try rolling the foam roller out on an angle away from the body.*
    - *For an even deeper release bend at the elbow and place the palms to the shoulders, with the foam roller under the elbow.*
    - *If unable to sit on your heels place a block or cushion between the heels to relax onto.*
    - *Get a partner and have them roll the acuball along the spine as you stretch with the foam roller.*

Benefits:
- o This is a great addition to the lat massage and may target more of the back muscles as a whole.
- o A good challenge for those with shortened front chest muscles and tightness in the under arm pocket.

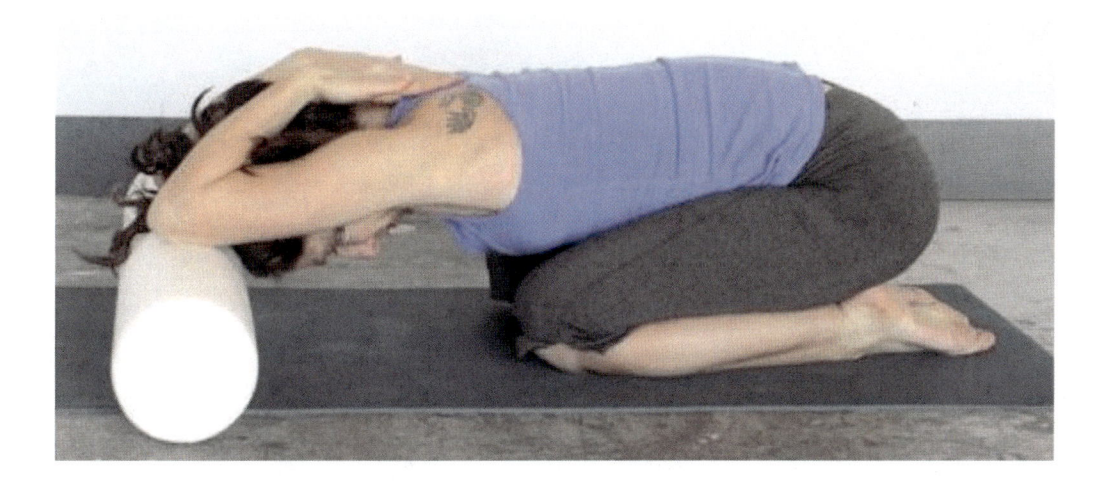

Camel (Lower Back Release)

To Begin:
- Come to your knees in a neutral position (like Tadasana) and place the foam roller behind you and latch hold with both arms palms facing inward.
- Exhale and draw upward on the pelvic floor to help keep the core strong and the back long.
- Inhale; gently begin to move the arms down the roller allowing the torso and pelvis to move forward pain free.
- Focus on allowing the hip sockets to gently without force shift slightly forward.
- Allow the arms to press into the foam roller to ensure it does not fall.
- Keep your core strong, and allow the tail-bone to point downward.
- Continue to breathe for up to ten breaths.
- Do not over extend in the neck; those with neck issues draw the chin to the chest (this will create a slightly different stretch along the spine).
- To come out, contract the pelvic floor and use your core to draw the body back to center, not the neck and head.
  - *Variations:*
    - *Try this standing in Tadasana as a standing back bend.*

Benefit:
- Here the chest is opened, abdomen, hip flexors, and quadriceps are stretched.
- The lower back is both massaged and released as the front of the pelvis is opened and stretched.
- Only go as far as the body will allow in its own timing.

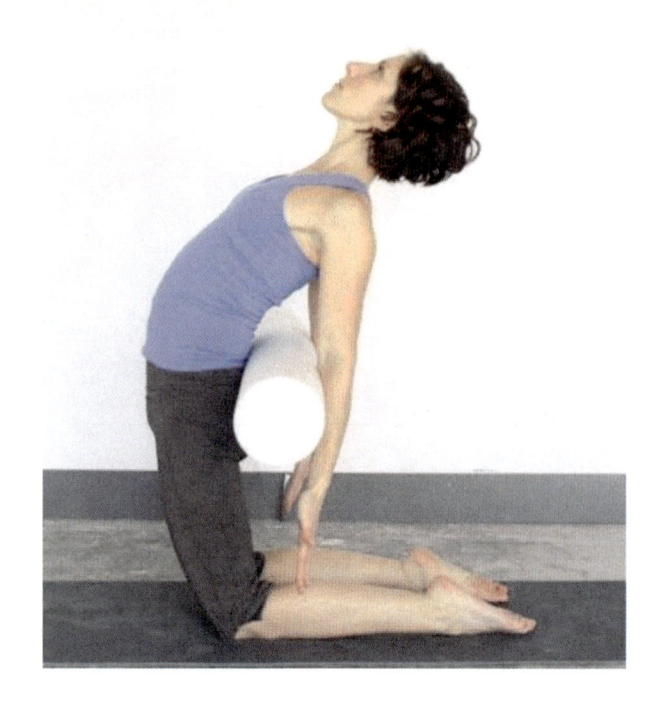

Gluteal Massage and Piriformis Release:

To Begin:
- Sitting on the foam roller lean onto your left gluteal and bend your right knee (the opposite knee) to help support and move the roller.
- Place both hands behind you on the floor elbows bent.
- Breathing calmly, and begin to roll on the buttock focusing on tender and tight areas of the body.
- Trigger point any areas of concern by holding on the foam roller, then beginning again with larger rolling motions.
- Work on each side for 2 to 5 minutes.
  - *Variations:*
    - *Lean up against the wall and place the acuball behind a gluteal muscle. Leaning into the acuBall begin to roll up and down the wall working to find any areas of tenderness. Trigger point any areas of concern and work until softness is achieved.*
    - *Figure for with the foam roller or acuBall under the glute.*

Benefits:
- Releasing the gluteus can give relief to the lower back and issues like sciatica.
- Restriction in the gluteus can cause SI joint instability as well as sacral and tail-bone misalignments even knee pain.
- Regular rolling can help improve yoga poses like Cow Face, Pigeon, and Lateral Angle.

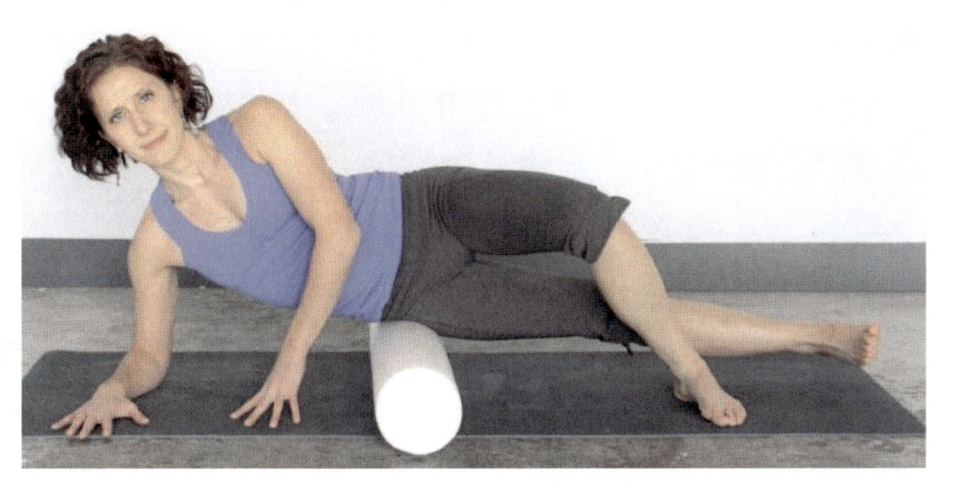

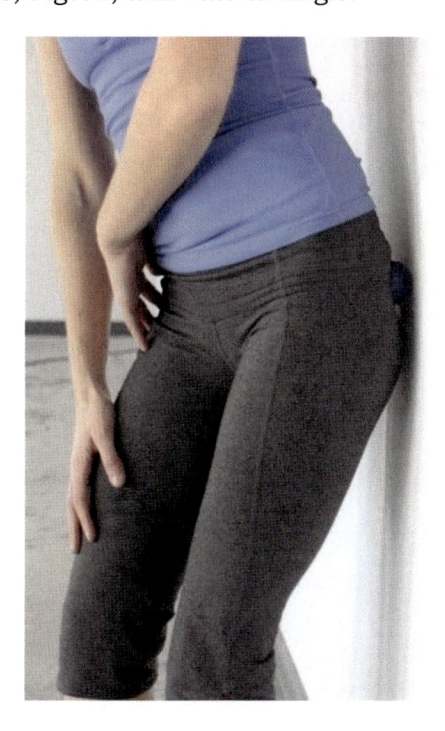

Sacral and Sacroiliac (SI) Joint Release:

To Begin:
- Lying down on your back, bend the knees and place the feet flat on the floor.
- Using the small acuBall place the ball under the sacrum and rest the pelvic girdle down onto the ball.
- Explore the sacrum, glutes and SI joints on each side of the tailbone as you rock and roll on the ball.
- Explore the ridge line of each side of the Ilium all the way down to the tailbone.
- Roll through the gluteus tissue and trigger point any area of tightness or restriction.
- Take one to five minutes rolling out the lower frame of the body.
    - *Variations:*
        - *Try this up against the wall.*

Benefits:
- Massaging the sacrum can help reset the sacral bones as well as helps to release the ligaments that attach to and from the sacrum and lower back.

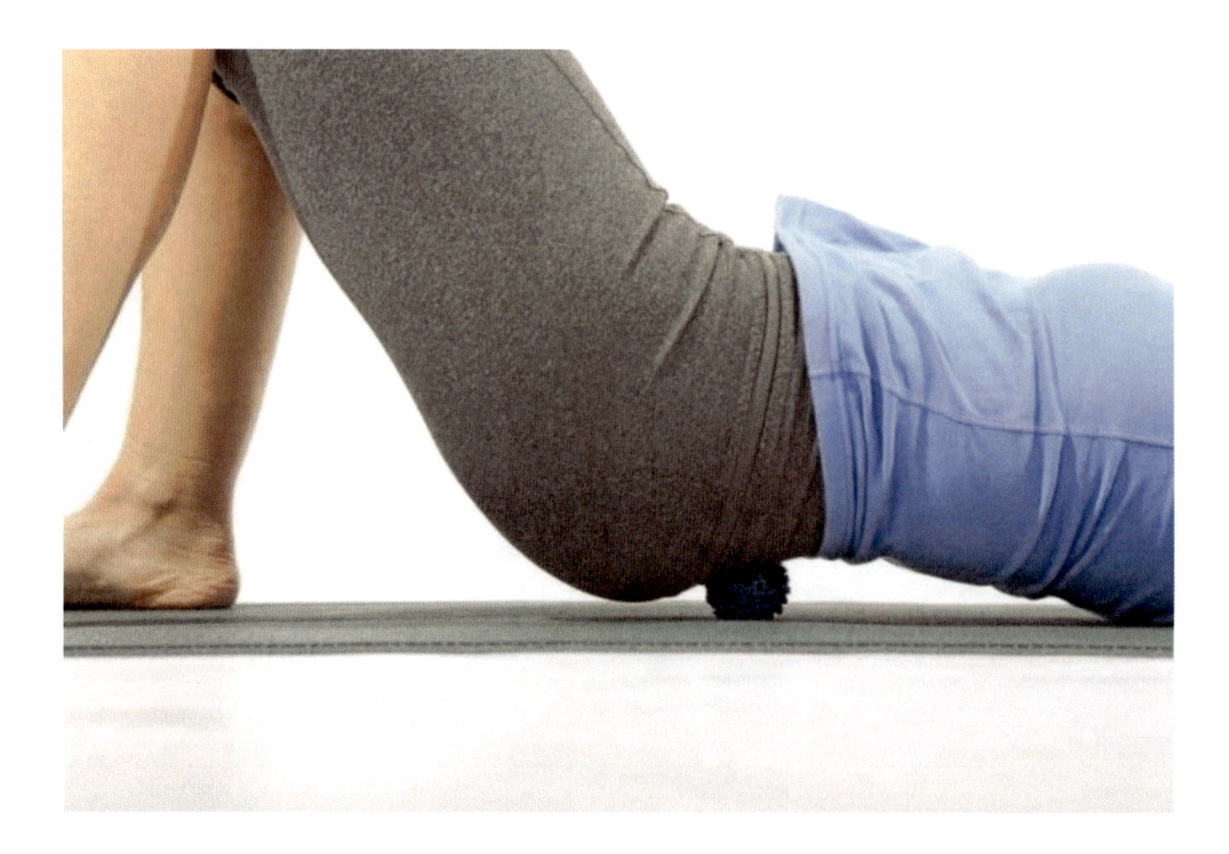

Figure Four (Hip Rotator Massage):

To Begin:
- Begin by sitting onto the foam roller, supporting your hands behind you.
- Cross the left ankle over the right knee and lean onto the left buttocks.
- Start by moving slowly and if the body will allow work your way up to larger movements, trigger point as needed.
- Continue to breathe slowly and deeply.
- Work on each side for 1 to 3 minutes.
  - *Variations:*
    - *For more of a challenge, work on this and place the right hand to the left knee (the crossed leg) and apply gentle pressure to increase the stretch and release.*
    - *Try this with the acuBall both on the floor and by leaning against the wall in the Figure Four Stretch position (see picture below).*
    - *For a gentler approach, extend the leg of the worked hip out straight on the floor.*

Benefits:
- By releasing the deep rotators of the hips, we allow more movement, flexibility and range of motion. This release will improve things like running, ease long-term sitting, practices like yoga as well as offer relief to aching hips.
- This is a great addition to yoga poses like pigeon, chair, and any other hip opener.

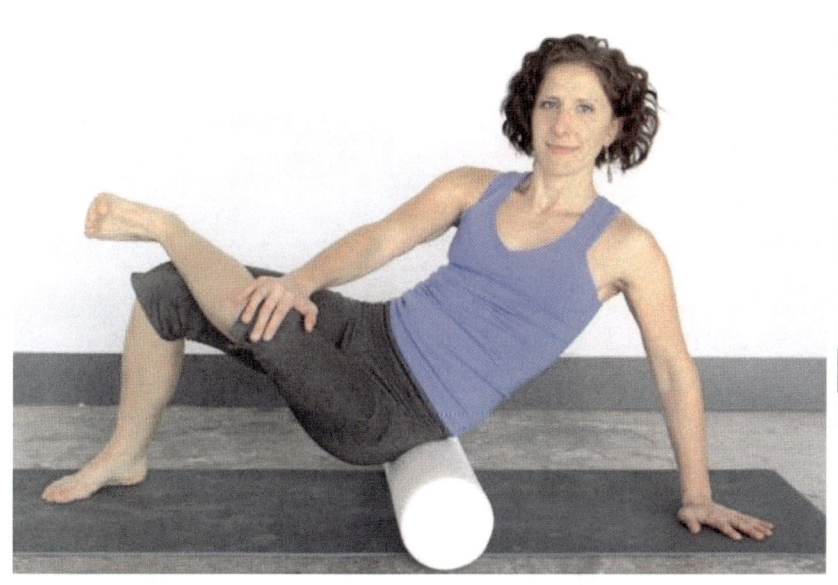

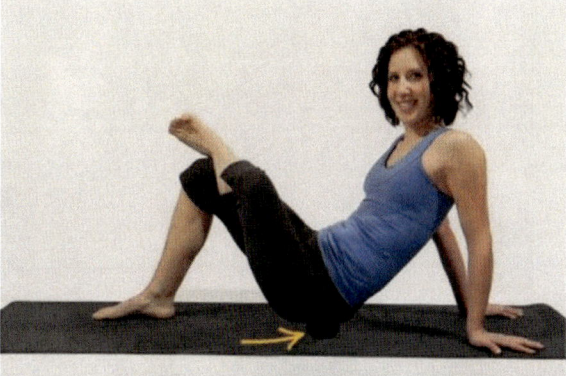

Adductor (Inner Thigh) Massage:

To Begin:
- Start by lying on your right side with the large acuBall in front of you
- Bend your left knee to a ninety-degree angle placing the inner thigh on the large acuBall.
- Using the support of your hands begin to slowly roll your inner thigh on the acuBall.
- Focusing on any areas of tenderness.
- Breathing deeply using the exhale to help release the body.
- Continue to work with this method for up to one minute.
- Repeat the opposite site.
  - *Variations:*
    - *Use a foam roller in place of a large acuBall.*
    - *Adjust the acuBall at any point on the inner leg, from knee to inner attachment sites at the hip.*

Benefits:
- This technique allows any restriction to dissolve and for someone with tight inner adductors.
- Those with knee pain (which is often a referred pain from the hip or ankle) may find relief.
- Remembering when we release tightness and restriction we have a better-increased range of motion.

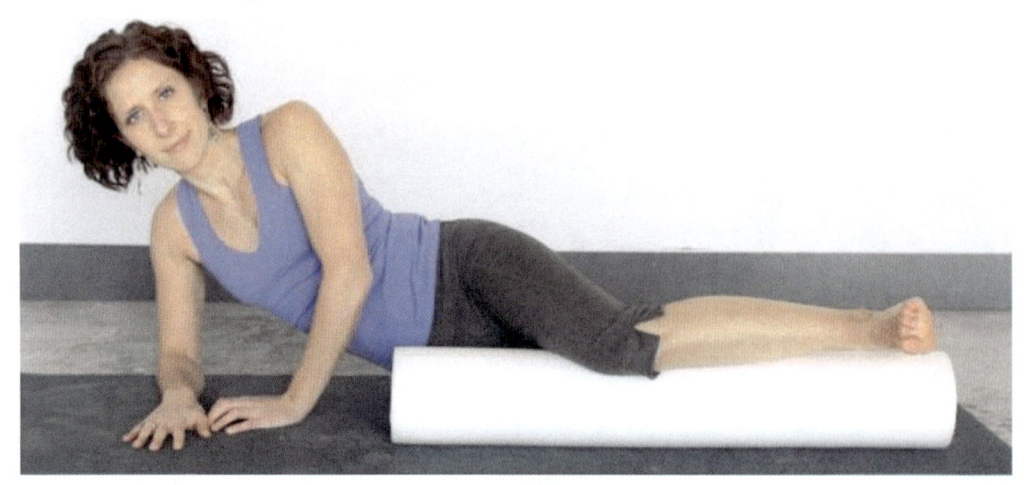

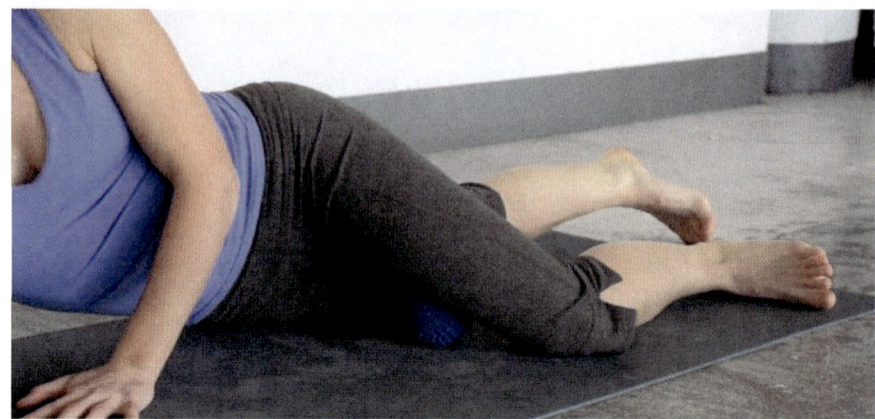

Hip Flexor Release Series:
Hip Flexor & Quadriceps Massage:

To Begin:
- ➢ Start by placing the foam roller on the floor crosswise underneath the hips.
- ➢ Rest the pelvis to the foam roller and the forearms to the floor for support.
- ➢ Using the arms to move the body forward and backward begin to slowly massage the hip flexors and quadriceps.
- ➢ Calmly breathing start to first focus on the hip flexors and work your way to the quadriceps, making larger rolling motions along the way.
- ➢ If one area is of more concern focus there for a while until tension dissolves.
- ➢ Try to roll the entire length of the muscle from top to bottom (hip to knee).
- ➢ Continue to roll for one to three minutes.
  - *Variations:*
    - *Solely focus on one hip flexor or one leg by leaning to one side or the other.*
    - *If there is a more restricted or tender side, return to that side for additional release.*
    - *Play with internal and external rotation of the legs to hit all angles of the quadriceps.*
    - *While rolling try bending the knees.*
    - *Play with internal and external rotation of the legs.*

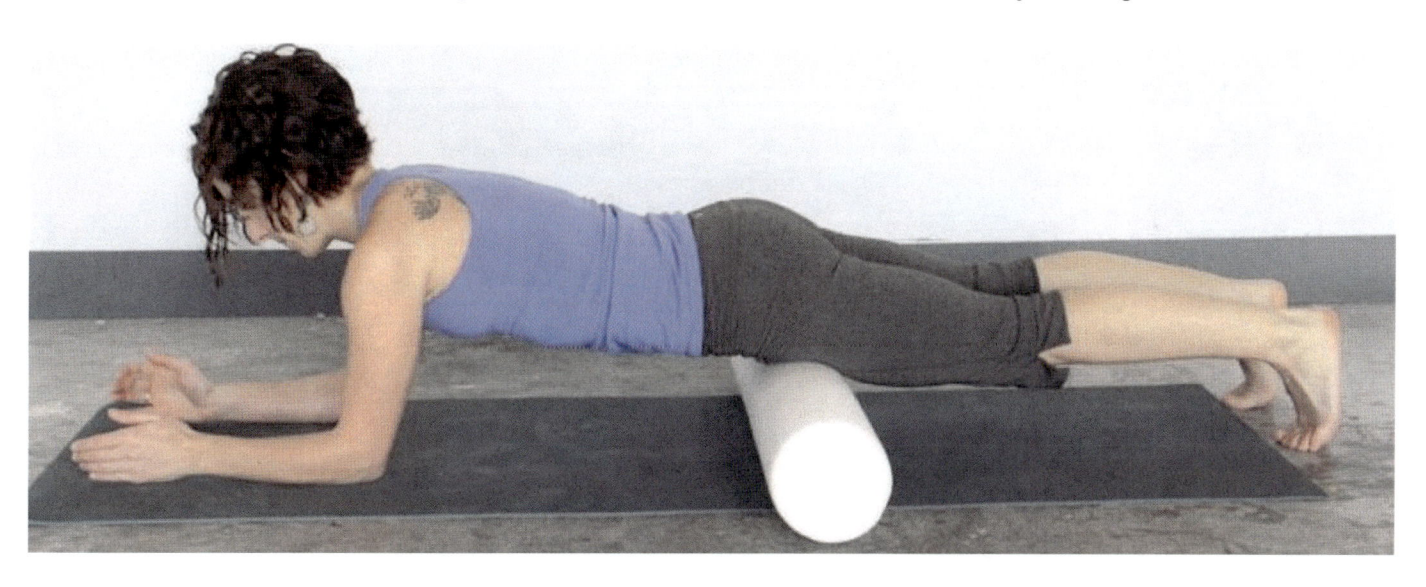

Hip Flexor Massage

Benefits:
- By releasing the hip flexors, the pelvis is released more effectively to neutral.
- For those with an anteriorly tilted pelvis (lordosis due to tight hip flexors and psoas), this is a very productive practice.
- Continuing to the quadriceps allows fascia to be released which can cause knee pain and even hip pain.
- Three of the (four) quadriceps attach at mid bone on the femur, so to massage those attachments can hopefully increase mobility and comfort.
- When the hamstrings are an issue, working on the opposite side of the body or the opposing muscle can sometimes offer more release than solely focusing on the area of issue.
- Releasing tension in the quads can help release the knee caps, which float in the tension of the thigh muscles.

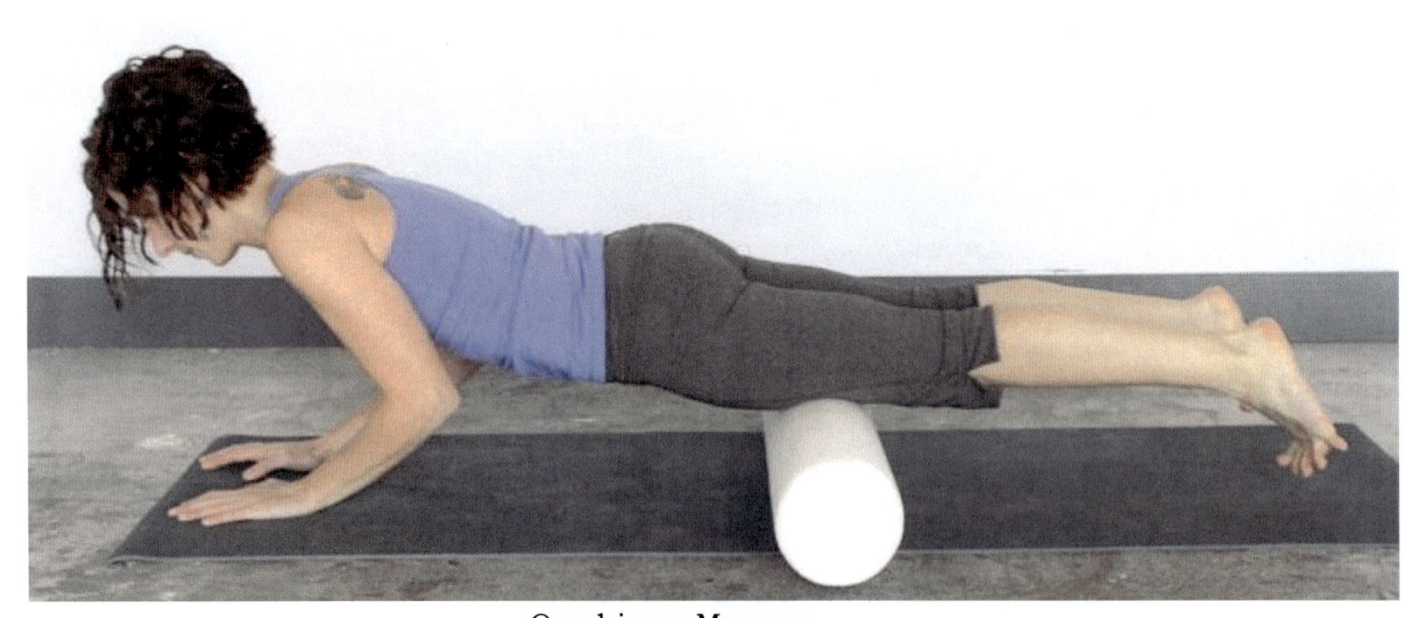

Quadriceps Massage

Supine Psoas Release

To Begin:
- Laying on your back, bend your knees to lift the hips and place the foam roller crosswise underneath your hip and sacrum area.
- Exhale, and slowly draw your left knee or thigh, and draw the leg into the chest.
- Inhale, work to reach through the lower leg by extending it outwards away from the body and simultaneously anchor it down into the floor.
- Focus more on drawing the femur (thigh bone) out of its hip socket rather than hugging the knee in.
- Move slowly and gradually hug the knee more deeply.
- Continue to hold this stretch for ten breaths to several minutes.
- There should be no pain or discomfort in the lower back (reassess your neutral or drop your hips down).
- Using core control and minimizing movement of the foam roller and not to let the lower back sag towards the floor, inhale, simultaneously switch the legs.
- Exhale, repeat the opposite side.
- Implement 2:1 ratio, revisiting the tighter groin a second time.
    - *Variations:*
        - *Omit the foam roller or any prop under the hip and lay flat on the floor.*
        - *Try this on the floor, a yoga block or a small ball to challenge the core even more.*
        - *Experiment moving the bent knee out away from the body still holding it with the hand.*
        - *To minimize the hip flexor stretch, bend up the lower leg.*
        - *Add in the acuball™ and massage the inner groin.*

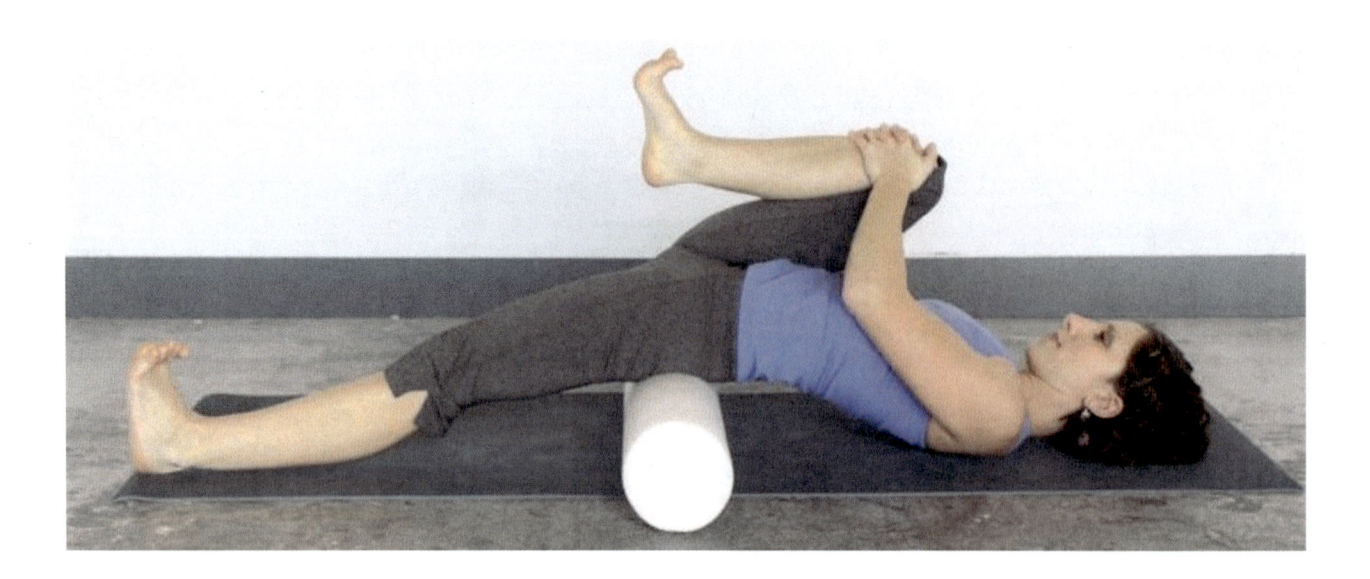

Benefits:
- By releasing the hip flexors, in particular the psoas, the pelvis is released more effectively to neutral.
- For those with an anteriorly tilted pelvis (lordosis due to tight hip flexors), this is a very productive practice.
- By gaining more length in the hip flexors the lower back will feel a greater release and decreased pain.
- This is a great anti-sitting release and a great practice for runners and bikers.

Prone Psoas and Ilicaus Release

To Begin:
- Lying on your abdomen, place the large acuBall above the left hip bone two fingers widths out from the navel (the point between the rectus abdominis and oblique).
- Start face down on the floor and slowly begin to rise up rocking to move the tissue around the acuball to find the posas muscle (will most likely feel tender).
- Using your feet work your body on top of the acuBall front and back releasing the deep muscles of the hip.
- Work on each side 10 breaths to several minutes, revisiting the more restricted side.
- Do not place the acuball lower than the ASIS (front hip bone) inside the pelvis.

Benefits:
- The psoas and hip flexor are a large area of interest for issues concerning the lower back. By working to release the hip flexors we allow more release in the lower back.
- Releasing the psoas can aid in more effective work with greater ease in accessing our deep core muscles.
- Psoas release for some can make all the difference in things like PMS cramping, digestive issues, and scar tissue.

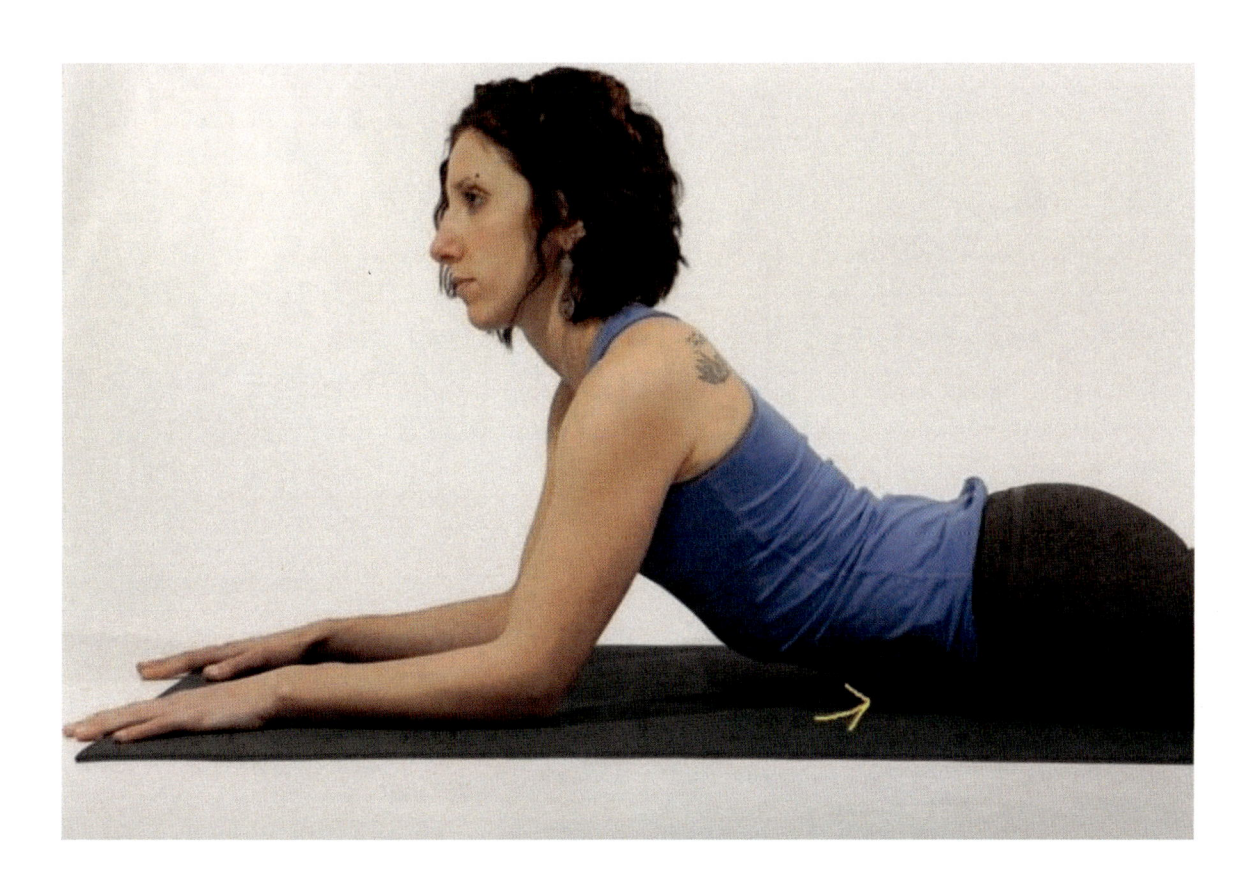

Groin Release in Bound Angle:

To Begin:
- Laying on your back draw the legs into a bound angle (or butterfly) position.
- Using the small acuBall, place the ball on top of the left inner hip.
- Applying appropriate pressure use your hand to move the ball through the groin's pelvic strings.
- Work to trace the ASIS point and make your way to releasing the pubis symphysis.
- Roll both above and on the pubis symphysis to help release the lower back.
- Work each hip as it needs to be for one to two minutes.
    - Variations:
        - Support the knees with blocks or rolled blankets if there is any knee strain.
        - Place the hips onto a block for more exposure to the groin.

Benefits:
- Releasing the groin and the pubis symphysis we are more able to release the lower back and pelvis back into neutral and work to a goal of pain free.
- It is common for women who have been pregnant to have pubis symphysis dysfunction, an issue in which the ligaments that keep the pubis bones in place to be pulling these two bones out of alignment. Regardless of pregnancy many however will benefit from this technique.

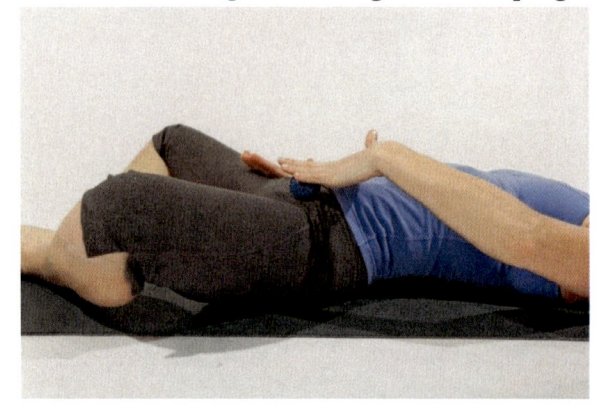

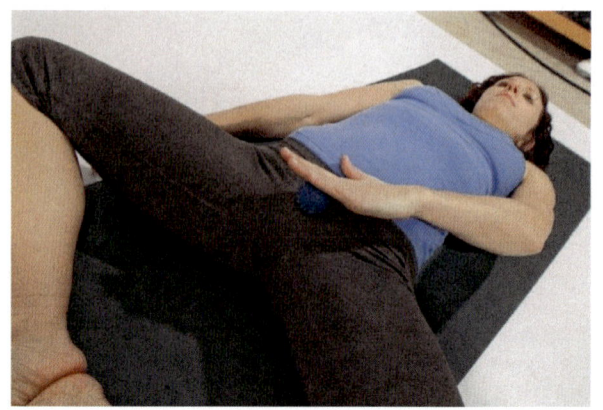

Iliotibal Band and Outer Thigh Massage:

To Begin:
- Lay to your outer left hip onto the center of the foam roller.
- Using the support of the left hand or forearm and right (top) foot placed in front of the lower leg begin to roll.
- Work the outer leg avoiding the outer knee and outer hip directly.
- Pause and trigger point areas of tenderness or restriction.
- Try to play with the angle of the body, allowing you to work the side of the leg from different angles.
- Continue to work here for one to two minutes and then repeat the opposite side.
- If you have a side of injury or deeper concern return to that side for additional release.
  - *Variations:*
    - *Standing against the wall place the large or small acuball between you and the wall. Begin to roll out the leg by moving up and down the wall adding only the amount of pressure your body can breathe through.*
    - *Try the large acuball on the floor as you did with the foam roller.*
    - *To make this more difficult while on the foam roller stack the legs on top of each other.*

Benefits:
- IT band and outer thigh restriction can cause foot, knee or hip pain.
- Extreme tightness here can cause misalignment in the pelvis and discomfort in simple things like walking.
- This is very common in runners and those that walk on the outer edges of the feet (called supination).

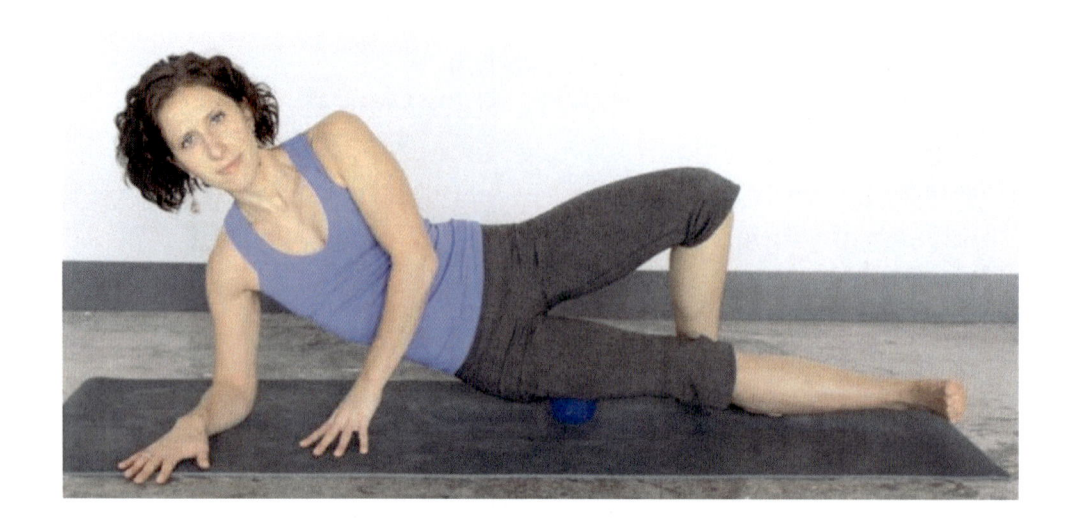

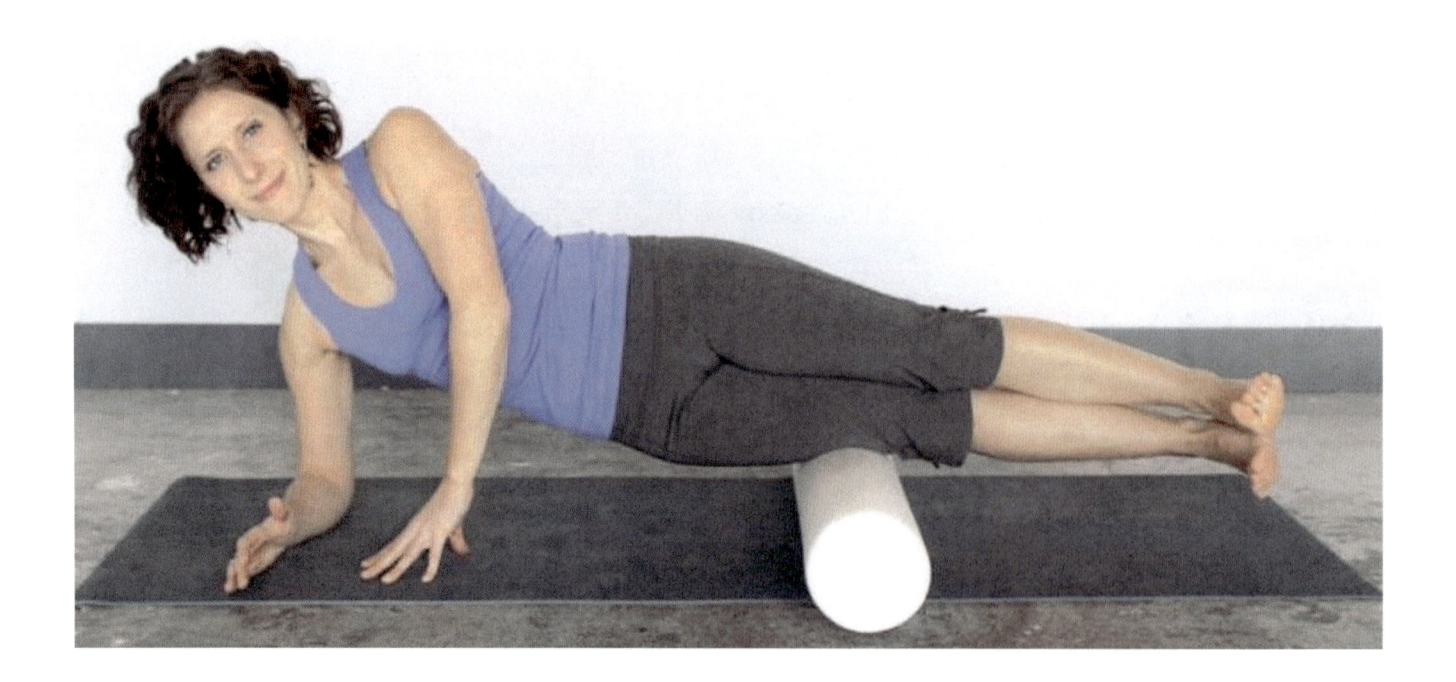

Outer Calf & Shin Massage:

To Begin:
- ➢ Start lying on your right side with the foam roller below the lower leg.
- ➢ Supported with the right forearm and sole of the left foot in front of the right knee begin to move allowing the roller to massage the outer calf.
- ➢ Making as large or small movements as the body will allow, breathe calmly and deeply.
- ➢ On and exhale keeping the core strong, turn the body placing both shins onto the foam roller and using the forearms roll out the shins.
- ➢ Inhale, open the body to the opposite side and begin to roll again.
- ➢ Spend 30 seconds to one minute on each area, going back to any area that was of greater concern.
    - o *Variations:*
        - *While rolling out the calf for more challenge keeping the oblique strong stack the legs and roll.*
        - *While on the shins, move from bent knees (table top) to a tucked position and back out again into a forearm like the plank. Remember to keep your core held tight.*
        - *Try any of these rolling methods by themselves.*
        - *Try any one of these rolling methods one leg at a time using the large acuBall.*
        - *Work singly from a seated position working on the calf with the foam roller or acuBall.*

Benefits:
- o This may assist with minimizing calf cramping releasing the fascia and also help with shin splints.
- o Restrictions in the lower leg can affect tibia and fibula alignment as well as affect the health of our feet and knees.

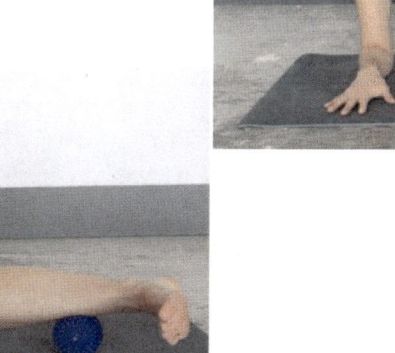

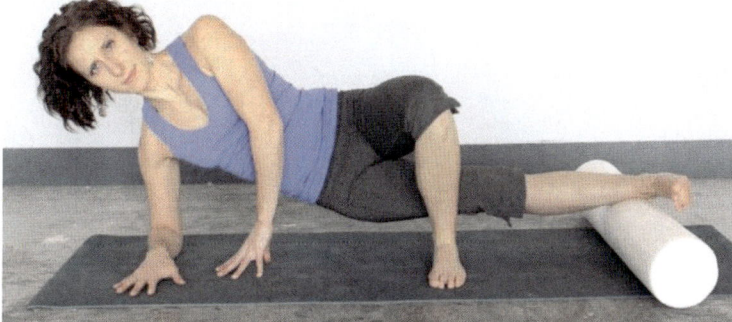

Hamstrings Massage:

To Begin:
- Place the foam roller underneath the hamstrings, with the hands placed comfortably behind you.
- Keeping the hips lifted slowly begin to roll the hamstrings along the foam roller.
- Playfully, experiment with moving the body shifting the focus for release on any of the four hamstring bodies.
- Gently roll up near the attachment sites at the sits bones and downward towards the lower half of the hamstring.
- If choosing to roll behind the knees, use the foam roller as the tissue is thinner at this part of the body.
- Continue to roll breathing calmly and deeply for up to two minutes.
  - *Variations:*
    - *To make this more intense cross the ankles or try lifting up one leg off the foam roller.*
    - *Try using the large acuBall working on one leg at a time on a smooth surface for easy gliding.*

Benefits:
- This can be a great way to help assist in releasing tight or restricted hamstrings; allowing more range of motion and less pain.
- Releasing the hamstrings increases the mobility of your back.
- Can aid in the release of pain in the knees and tension in the lower leg.

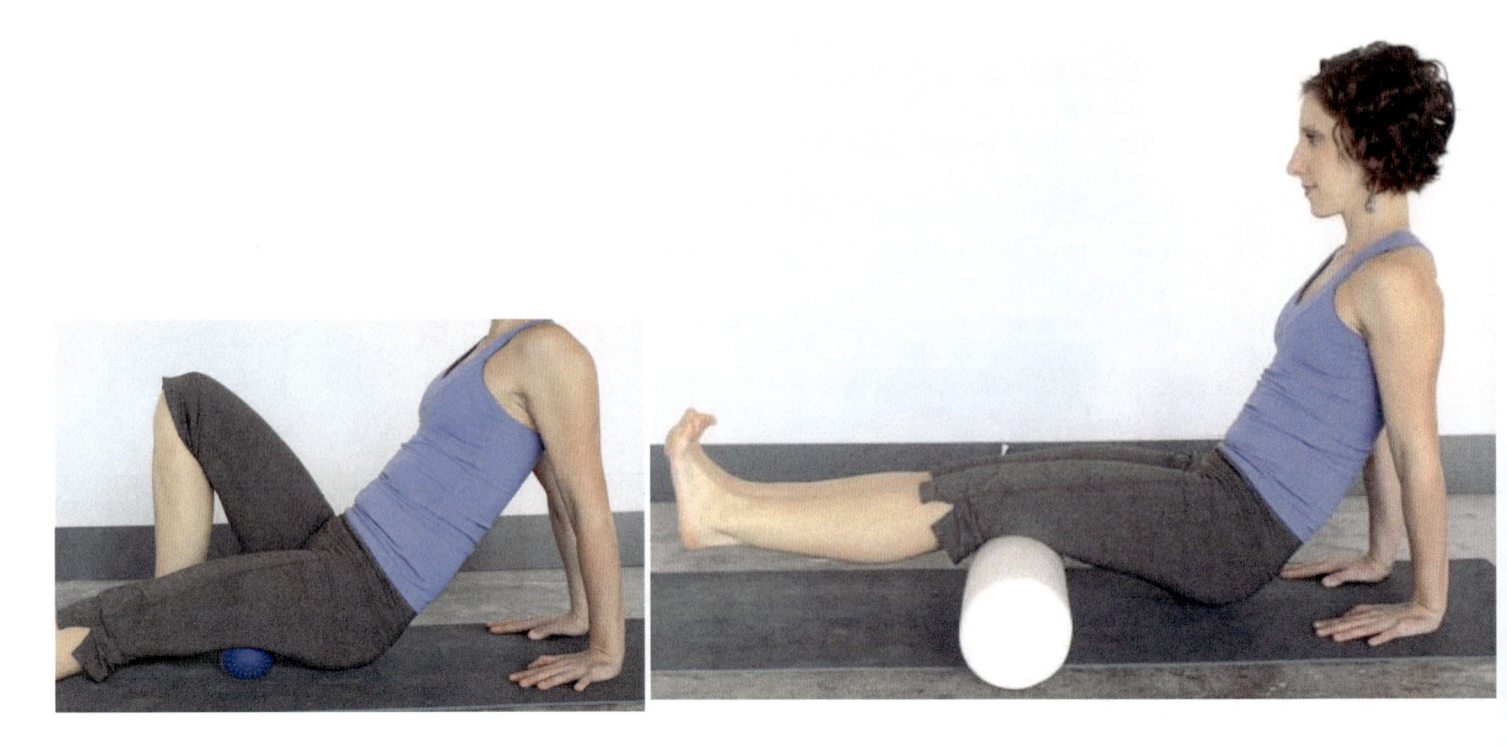

Foam Roller Arm Series:
Arm Scissors and Arm Extension:

To Begin:
- ➢ Lying on the foam roller in neutral activate the pelvic floor.
- ➢ Bring the arms up to hip level hovering over the floor alongside the body, palms face in.
- ➢ Keeping neutral and using the core to keep the body stable.
- ➢ INHALE steadily reach the right arm up and over alongside the right ear.
- ➢ Notice if the ribs pop or if the body rolls out of alignment. Only reach the arm as far as the body can support neutral.
- ➢ EXHALE and simultaneously switch the arms, reaching the left alongside the ear and the right next to the body.
- ➢ Be conscious to keep the movement only in the shoulder, and not in the torso.
- ➢ Continue with this mindful-movement for up to a minute.
  - *Variation: Now try moving both arms simultaneously up and alongside the ears.*
  - *If extending the arms on an inhale is too difficult, try it on an exhale and work up to an Inhalation.*
  - *Try this with hand weights*
  - *For more core stability try this with a small ball or yoga block between the thighs.*

Benefits:
- An effective practice of stability and mobility, the shoulders and muscles that support the shoulders are both stretched and strengthened.
- A great practice for rib thrusters, or instability in the shoulder girdle.
- A simple yet effective practice to build up better core stability and health.

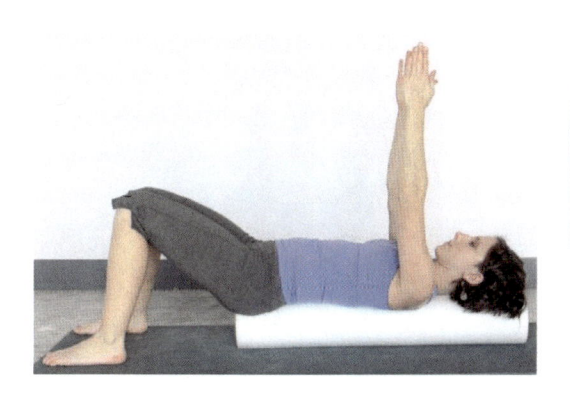

Double Arm Phase 1: Exhale

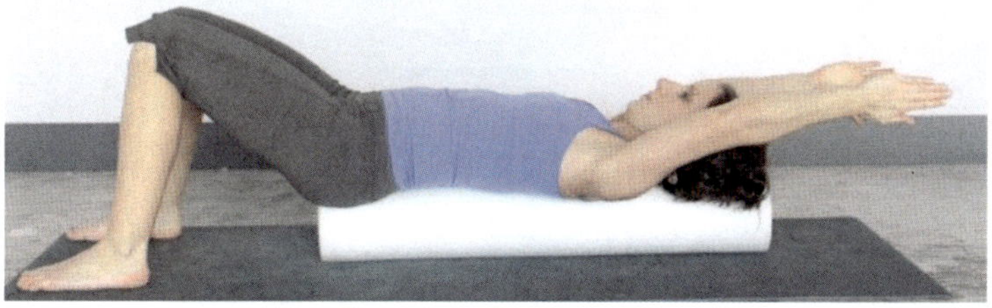

Upper: Double Arm Phase 2: Inhale / Lower: Single Arm

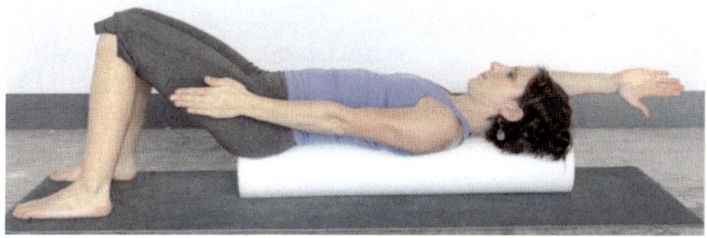

Foam Roller Arm Series:
Arm Circles:

To Begin:
- Lying on the foam roller in neutral and activate the pelvic floor.
- INHALE; raise the arms up vertical towards the ceiling, palms face in.
- EXHALE, find a steady body position.
- INHALE; extend the arms overhead alongside the ears no lower than the ears, palms face in.
- Turning the palms to face up begin to as the arms move to "T".
- EXHALE, palms turn in towards the body as they move alongside the hips level with the foam roller.
- At the edge of the exhale swipe the arms vertical back to where they started, making a circle with the arms moving from the shoulder.
- Really pay attention to if the movement is coming from the shoulder or the upper back.
- Continue with the movement for up to one minute.
  - *Variations:*
    - *Try this with light hand weights*
    - *For more support place a small ball or yoga block between the thighs to help the pelvic floor engage.*

Benefit:
- This can enhance range of motion (ROM) in the shoulders and help with rotator issues and restriction. Here the chest muscles are stretched equally to the muscles of the upper back and under arm.

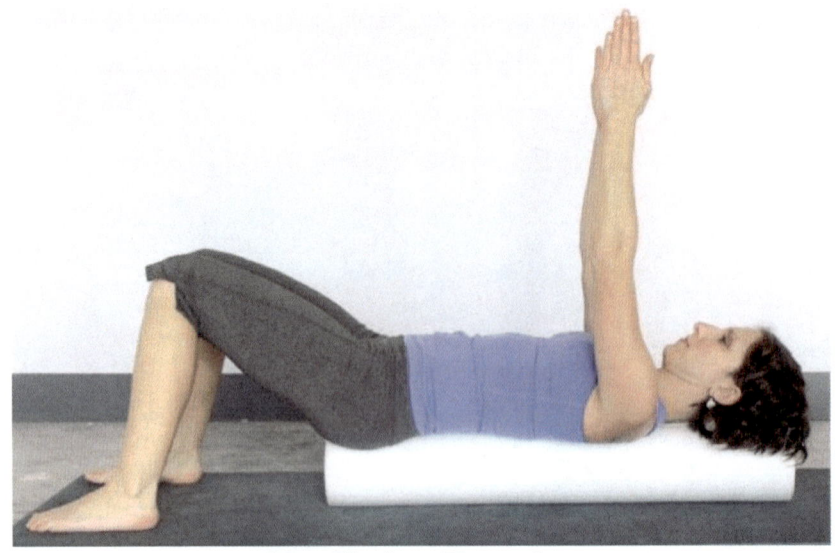

Arm Circles: Phase 1

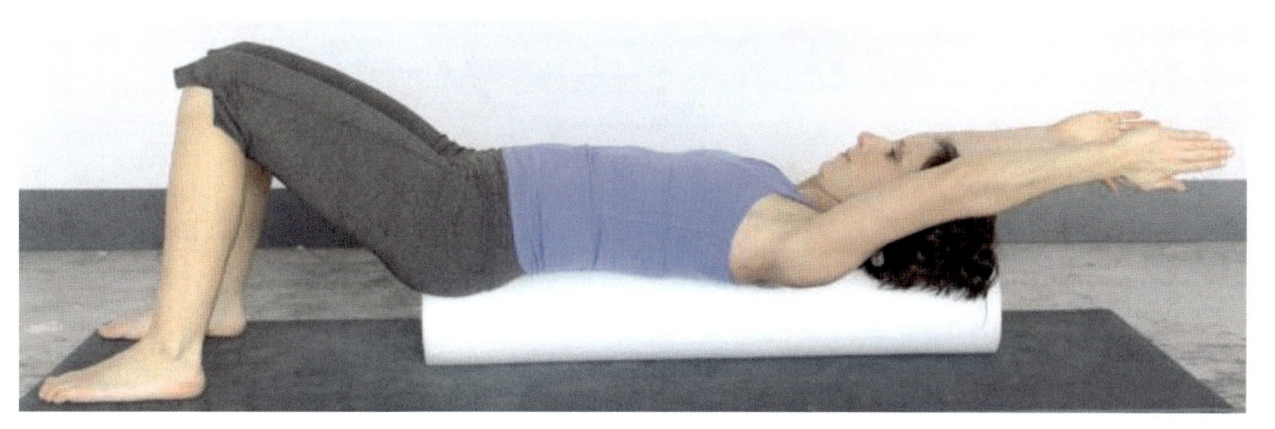

Arm Circles: Phase 2

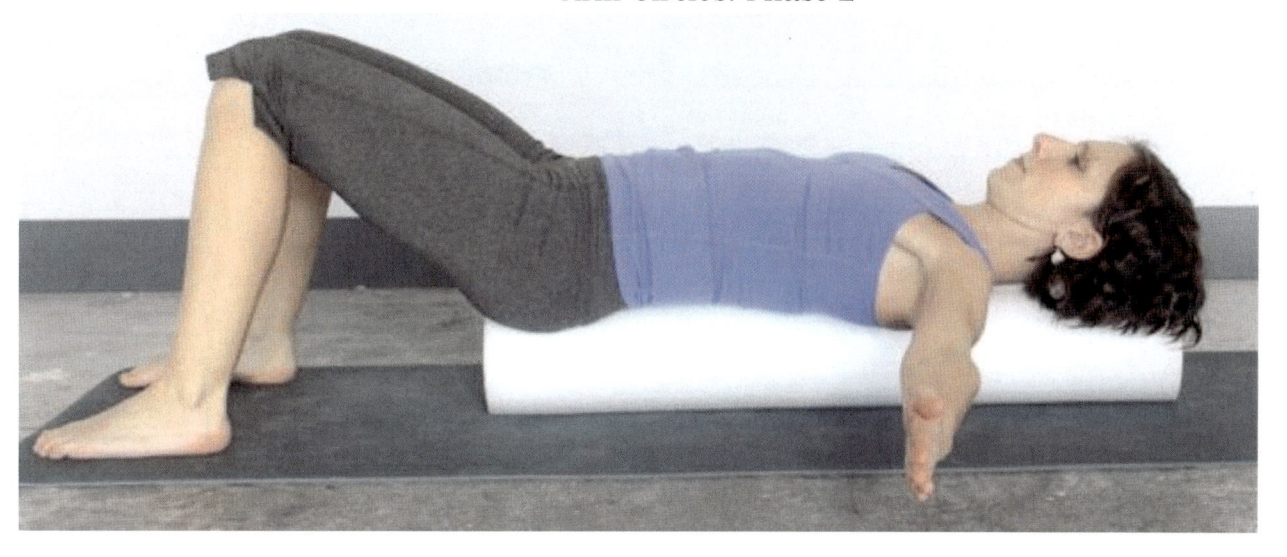

Arm Circles: Phase 3

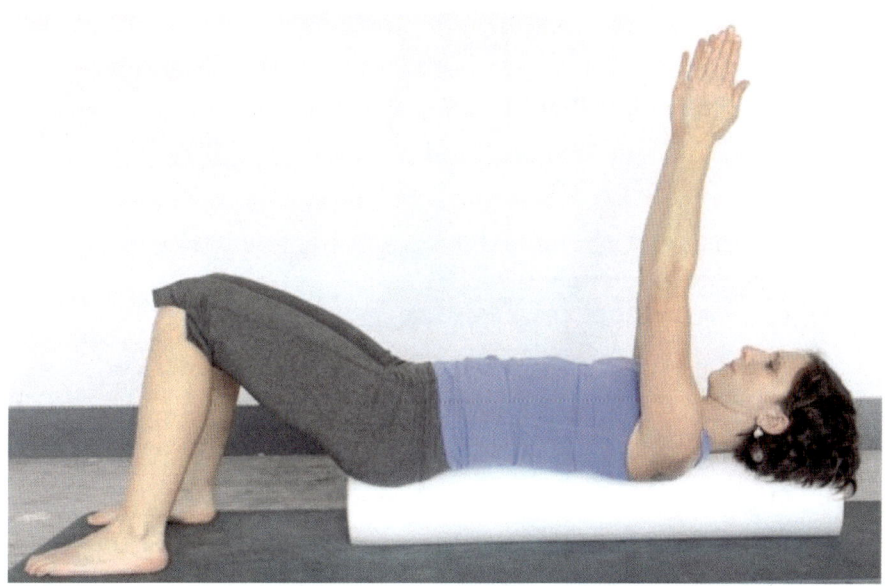

Arm Circles: Phase 4

Foam Roller Arm Series:
Deltoid Fly:

To Begin:
- Lying on your foam roller align the feet beneath the hips at a comfortable distance from the foam roller and find neutral and activate the pelvic floor.
- Extend both arms out to a "T" position, off the floor, hovering in neutral with the shoulder.
- INHALE, to prepare for the movement holding at "T", *palms and elbow folds facing upward with a slight bend in the elbow.*
- EXHALE; slide the arms towards the hips keeping level with the shoulder line.
- INHALE, return to a "T" position being careful to not travel above the shoulder.
- Remember to keep a strong core and the shoulders level, trying not to hunch the upper body.
- Keeping stable on the foam roller, slow the movement or release the weights if you are unable to stay stable on the foam roller.
- Repeat this movement, 8-12 times, slow and steady.
    - *Variations:*
        - *Place a small ball or yoga block between the thighs to help keep the core active.*
        - *Release the weights and perform this movement.*
        - *Try performing this movement with one foot off the floor and then try the other, notice which side is more stable. Implement the 2:1 ratio towards the weaker side.*
        - *Also, try this with the palms facing downward and inward.*

Benefits:
- Shoulders are released and the shoulder girdle is stabilized.
- Building lean muscle around the shoulder joints is a healthy way to prevent shoulder injury.
- Jerky, unstable, mindless movements or movements with too much weight are unhealthy and could cause injury.
- Muscles primarily worked but not limited too are the deltoids, triceps, subscapularis (inner arm pit) and infraspinatus (outer wing of the upper shoulder (scapula).

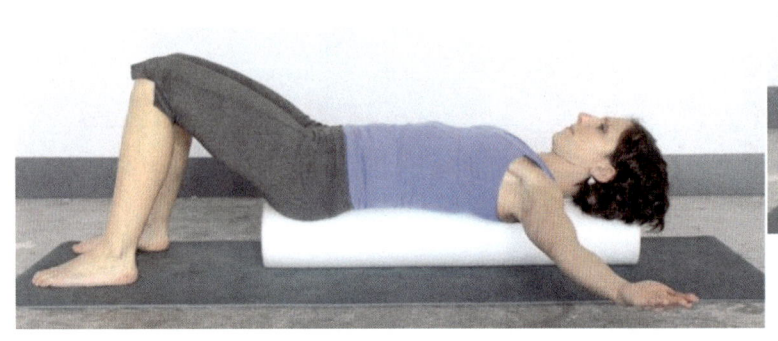

Left: Phase 1: Inhale / Upper: Phase 2: Exhale

Foam Roller Arm Series:
Pectoral and Biceps Curl:

To Begin:
- ➢ Lying on your foam roller align the feet beneath the hips at a comfortable distance from the foam roller and find neutral.
- ➢ Extend both arms out to a "T" position, off the floor, neutral with the shoulder.
- ➢ INHALE, to prepare for the movement holding at "T".
- ➢ EXHALE; bending from the elbow fold the arm in towards the chest.
- ➢ Always make sure you honor a one degree bend in the elbow not to overextend in the joint.
- ➢ INHALE, return to a "T" position.
- ➢ Remember to keep a strong core and the shoulders level, trying not to hunch the upper body.
- ➢ Repeat this movement, 8-12 times, slow and steady.
  - o *Variations:*
    - *Try this with light hand weights.*
    - *Place a small ball, yoga block or large acuball™ between the thighs to help keep the core active.*
    - *Try performing this movement with one foot off the floor and then try the other, notice which side is more stable. Implement the 2:1 ratio towards the weaker side.*
    - *Try this movement traveling above the shoulder, watch not to shrug the shoulders or round the upper body. This is not an option for someone with a rotator injury or shoulder issues.*
      - *Inhale to extend overhead and Exhale to float to the hips.*

Benefits:
- o Here the shoulders and chest muscles are worked and the shoulder girdle is stabilized.
- o Building lean muscle around the shoulder joints is a healthy way to prevent shoulder injury.
- o Jerky, unstable, mindless movements or movements with too much weight are unhealthy and could cause injury.
- o Muscles primarily worked but not limited too are the deltoids, biceps, pectoralis major and minor, subscapularis (inner arm pit, muscle of the rotator) and serratus anterior (muscles covering outer lateral portion of the rib cage).
- o Working with the foam roller encourages openness in the chest, essential when working with this type of exercise.

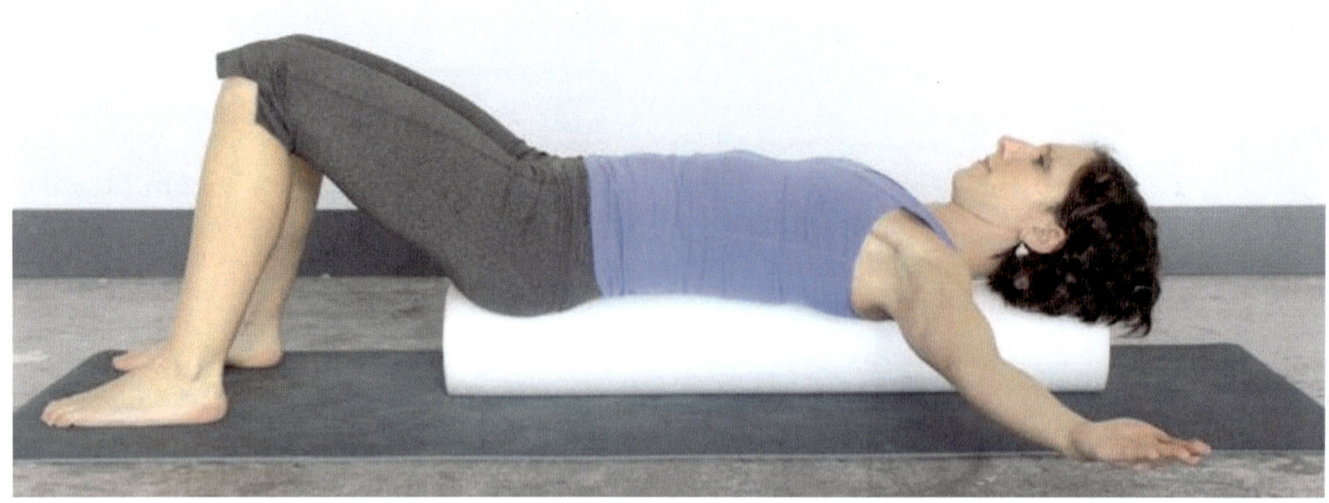

Bicep Curl Phase 1: Inhale

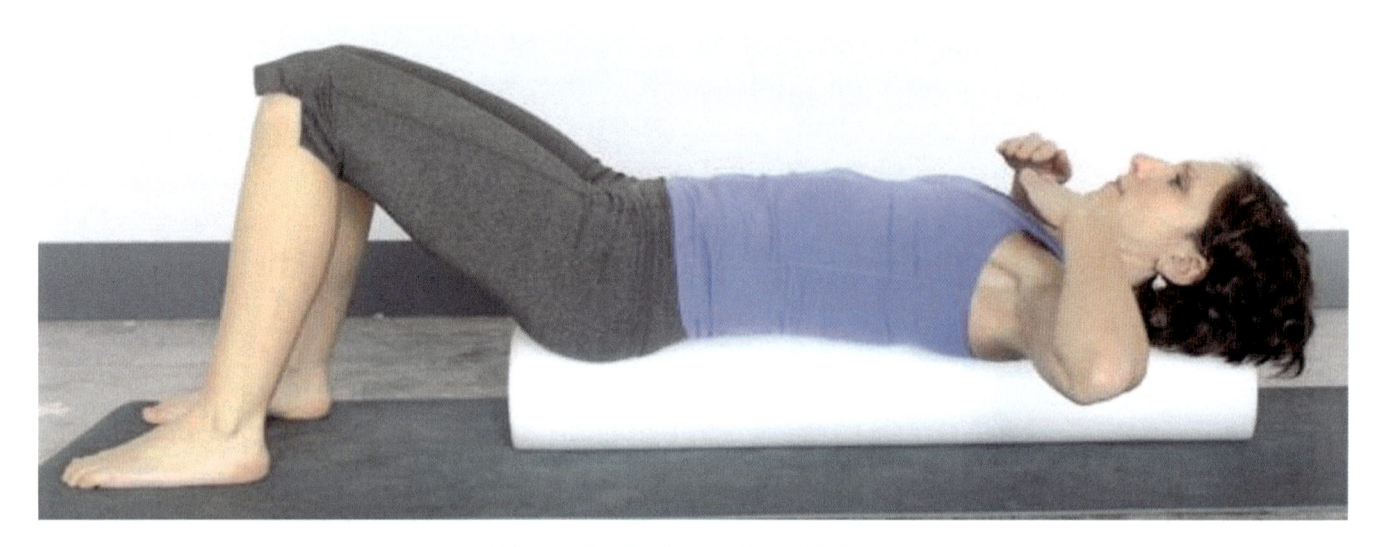

Bicep Curl Phase 2: Exhale

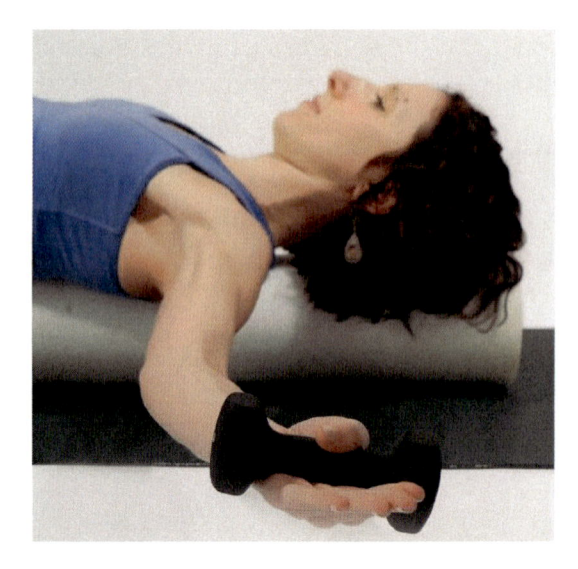

Phase 1: With weights

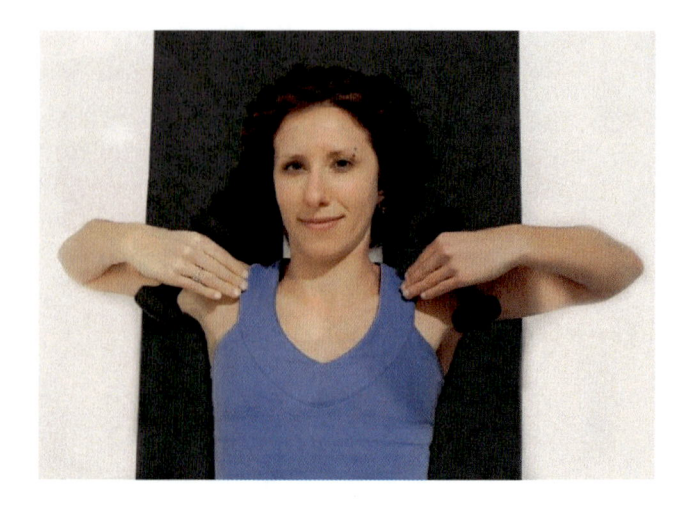

Phase 2: With weights

Foam Roller Arm Series:
Basic Triceps Extension:

To Begin:
- ➢ Lying on the foam roller in neutral pelvis and spine, feet a comfortable distance away from the roller at hips' width.
- ➢ Lift the arms up to the sky, wrist above the shoulder and interlace the fingers or hold a yoga block.
- ➢ Keep the folds of the elbows facing inward and slightly towards you, pay attention if they try to rotate to extend.
- ➢ Keeping neutral in the shoulder girdle and rib cage.
- ➢ INHALE, work to breathe laterally and starting with a slight bend in the elbows, extend the arms over head no further than roller height.
- ➢ Be mindful to only move as far as the shoulder will allow (don't take the ribs with).
- ➢ Imagine dipping the weights or your hands in a small cup of water almost out of reach.
- ➢ EXHALE; powerfully lift the weights using your core back up to starting.
- ➢ Repeat this movement 8-12 times.
  - *Variations:*
    - *Use light hand weights or a yoga block, held together by both hands.*
    - *Place a small ball or yoga block between the thighs to help keep the core active.*
    - *Try performing this movement with one foot off the floor and then try the other, notice which side is more stable.*
  - *Advanced Variations:*
    - *1: Exhale, steadily lift one leg and bring the weights towards the leg (no movement on the roller), Inhale release and repeat the opposite side.*
    - *2: Exhale, peel the head and upper torso off the foam roller and glide the weights towards the stable knees, Inhale release the head and spine arms to the ceiling or alongside the ears. Be careful not to round the upper torso when lifting.*

Benefits:
- Here the core is worked and all the muscles of the spine active.
- The triceps and muscles of the rotator cuff are both stretched and strengthened.
- Holding a block or weight in the hands can offer support and enhance the stretch.
- A great release in the shoulder girdle and under arm.

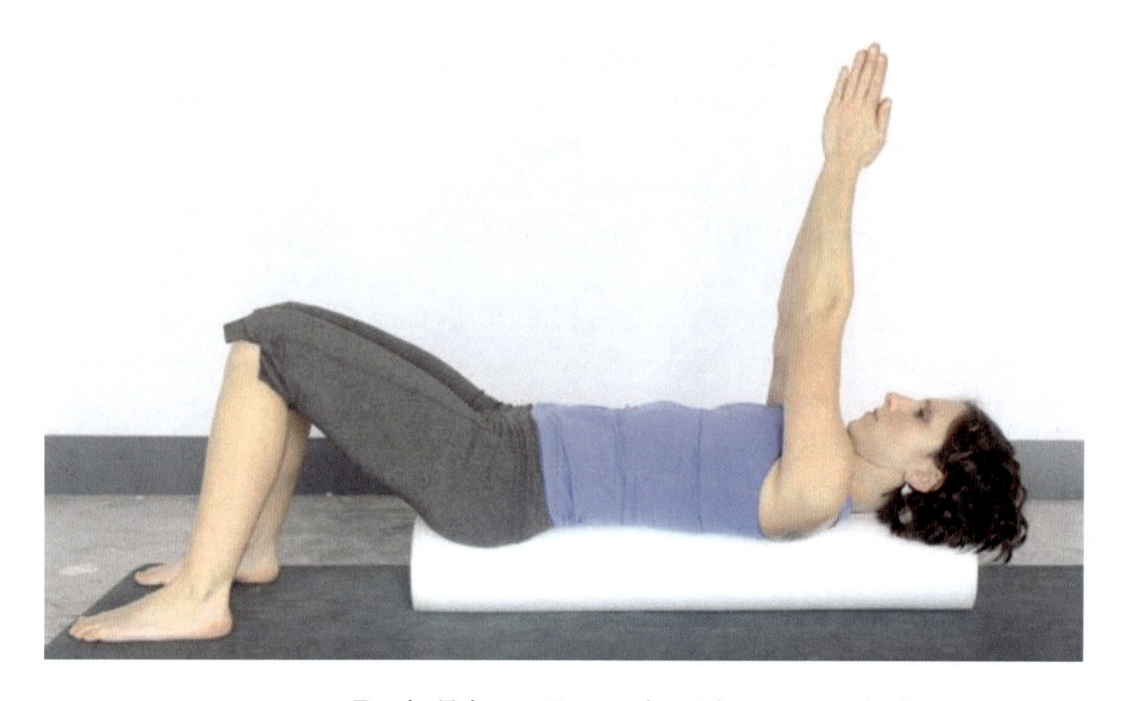

Basic Triceps Extension Phase 1: Exhale

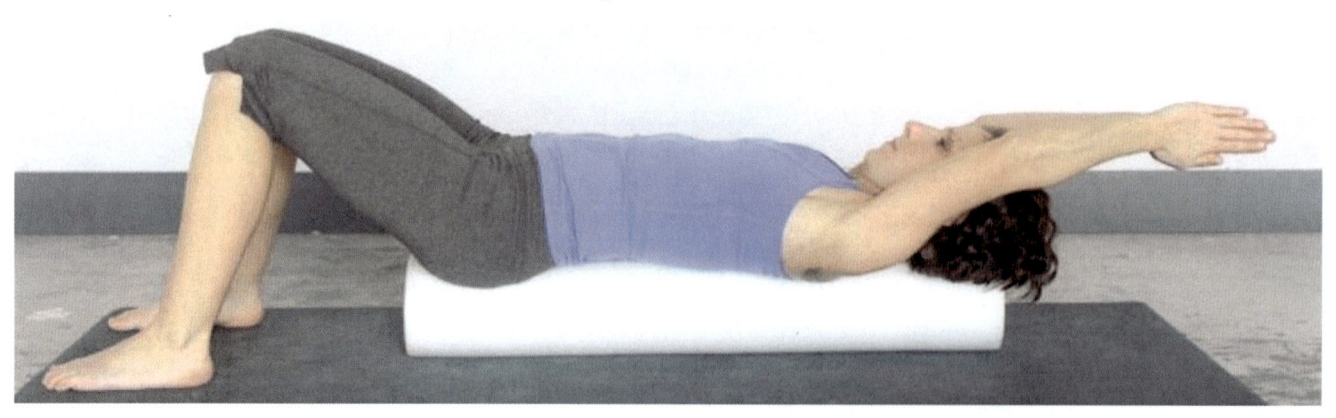

Basic Triceps Extension Phase 2: Inhale

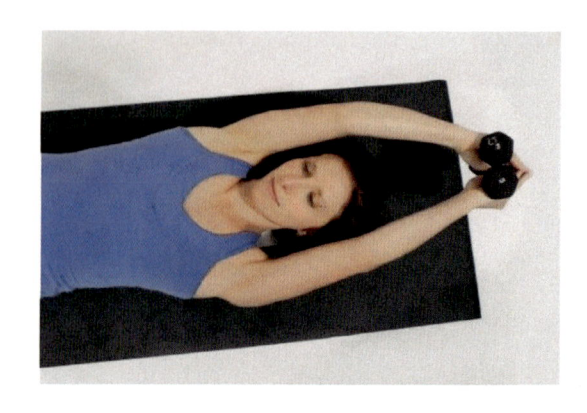

Right: With weights

Foam Roller Arm Series:
Weighted Triceps Extension with Heel Drop:

To Begin:
- Lying on the foam roller in neutral pelvis and spine, feet a comfortable distance away from the roller at hips' width.
- Lift the arms up to the sky, wrist above the shoulder hold your weight with the fingers interlaced or both hands on the weight.
- Keep the folds of the elbows facing inward and slightly towards you, pay attention if they try to rotate to extend.
- Work to keep neutral in the shoulder girdle and rib cage.
- EXHALE and lift the right leg up to a table top (shin parallel with the ceiling and foot flexed).
- INHALE and work to breathe laterally and extend the arms with weights overhead (initiating with a slight bend in the elbows to help release the shoulders) as you extend the floating heel down towards the floor, no further than roller height.
- Be mindful to only move as far as the shoulder will allow (don't take the ribs with) and core will keep you stable (no arching in the lower back).
- Imagine dipping the weights or your hands in a small cup of water almost out of reach.
- EXHALE; powerfully lift the weight along with your floating leg, using your core, back up to starting (your joints are not pulling the limbs back up, your core is).
- Repeat this movement 8-12 times or for one minute.
  - *Variations:*
    - *Omit the weight.*
    - *Only work the upper body, keeping both feet on the mat.*
    - *Use a weight from one pound to eight pounds, there should be no stress on the shoulders.*

Benefits:
- Here the core is worked and all the muscles of the spine active.
- The triceps, muscles of the rotator cuff, and upper back are both stretched and strengthened.
- A great release in the shoulder girdle and under arm is achieved with proper alignment.
- Deep core and legs are toned when combine with the upper body movement.

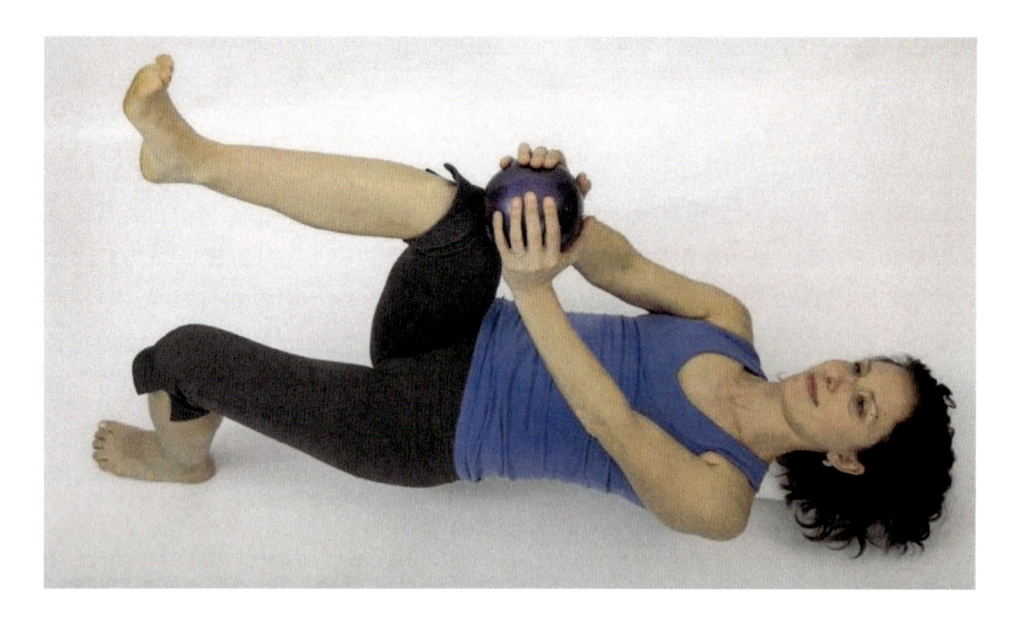

Weighted Triceps: Phase 1: Exhale

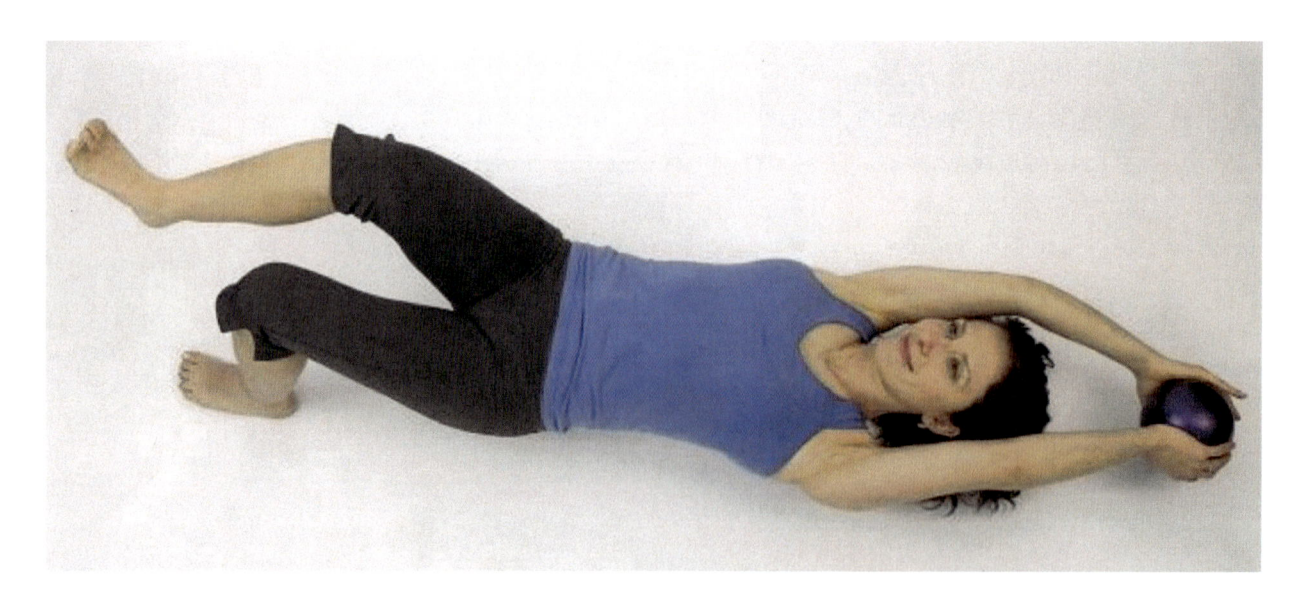

Weighted Triceps: Phase 2: Inhale

Foam Roller Arm Series:
Weighted Triceps Extension with Core Flexion:

To Begin:
- Lying on the foam roller in neutral pelvis and spine, feet a comfortable distance away from the roller at hips' width.
- Lift the arms up to the sky, wrist above the shoulder hold your weight(s) with the fingers interlaced or both hands on the weight.
- Keep the folds of the elbows facing inward and slightly towards you, pay attention if they try to rotate to extend.
- Work to keep neutral in the shoulder girdle and rib cage.
- INHALE and work to breathe laterally and initiating with a slight bend in the elbows, extend the arms and weight(s) overhead, no further than roller height (only extend the arms as far as you can keep from flaring the front lower ribs).
- Be mindful to only move as far as the shoulder will allow (don't take the ribs with) and core will keep you stable (no arching in the lower back).
- Imagine dipping the weights or your hands in a small cup of water almost out of reach.
- EXHALE and begin to lift the weight, when the weight is just above the head begin to roll the upper back off the foam roller (relax the shoulders as you do) being sure to use your upper abdominals and deep core not your neck and chest muscles (no strain).
- Repeat this movement 8-12 times or for one minute.
    - *Variations:*
        - *Omit the weight.*
        - *Don't extend the arms alongside the ears.*
        - *Use a weight from one pound to eight pounds, there should be no stress on the shoulders*

Benefits:
- Here the core is worked and all the muscles of the spine active.
- The triceps, muscles of the rotator cuff, and upper back are both stretched and strengthened.
- A great release in the shoulder girdle and under arm is achieved with proper alignment.
- There is an emphasis on the upper abdominals and rectus abdominis here (if you can keep from flaring the rib cage).
- Neck pain is a sure sign the upper abdominals are not firing properly and thus the neck is trying to do all the work, consider omitting the half curl up.

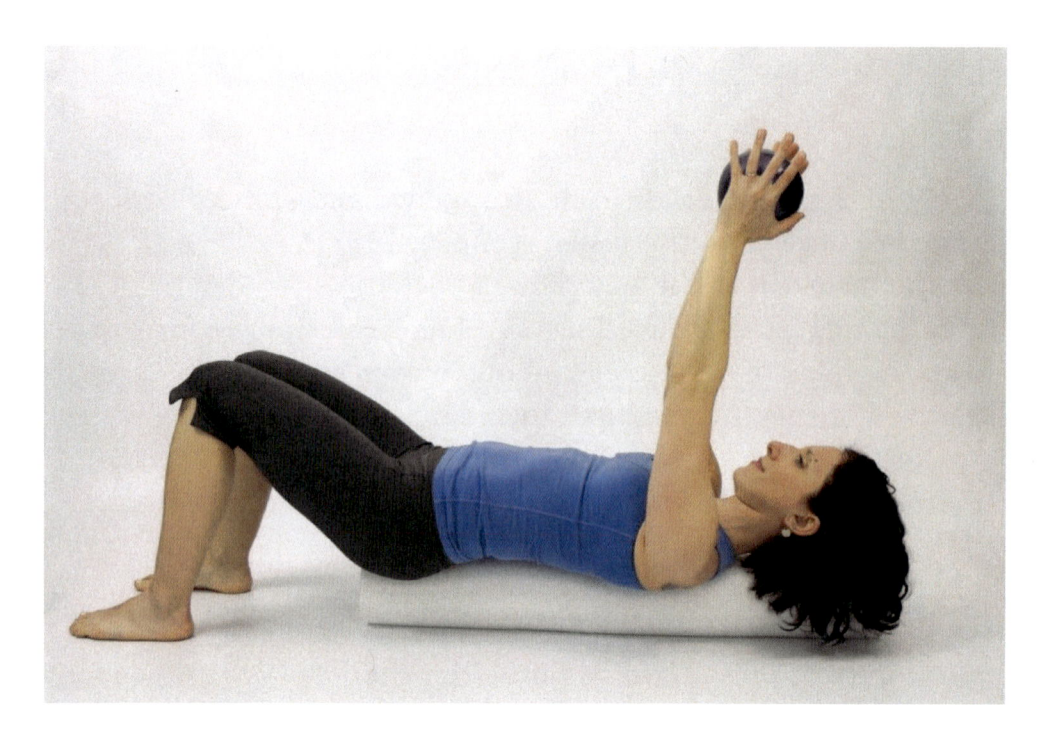

Core Flexion Phase 1: Inhale

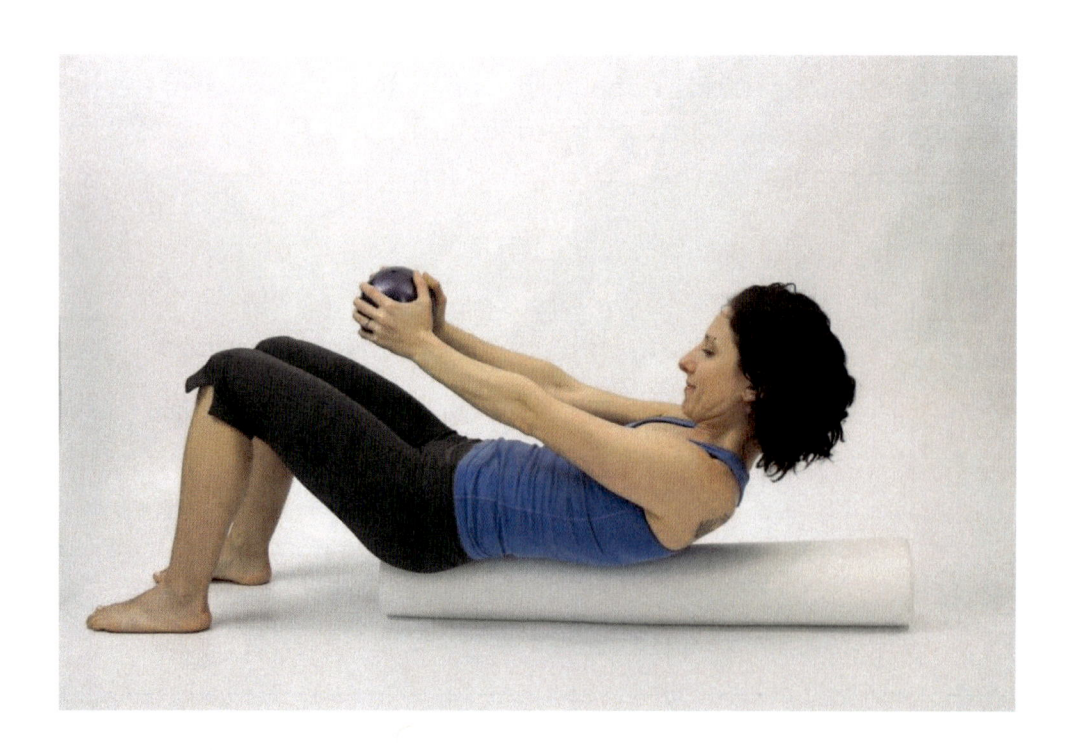

Core Flexion Phase 2: Exhale

Supine Stabilization Series:
Basic Leg Extension:

To Begin:
- ➢ Lying on the foam roller feet at a hips distance and the entire spine supported on the roller in neutral, place a small ball or yoga block between the knees. Choose any hand and arm option.
- ➢ INHALE to prepare for movement.
- ➢ EXHALE and engage the inner thighs and contract the core region, creating stability on the roller.
- ➢ INHALE to lift and extend the right leg 45° keeping the inner knees together.
- ➢ EXHALE pause extended feeling very stable and solid.
- ➢ INHALE to return the foot the floor and EXHALE pause at center.
- ➢ Repeat this series 5-8 times on each side. Working to be as stable as possible limiting any rocking and swaying.
  - o *Variations:*
    - *Place a block, a small ball, or large acuBall between the knees.*
    - *Keep the knees together but lift the leg where the shin is parallel with the ceiling only (table top).*
    - *To make this harder extend the arms upwards towards the sky palms face in.*
  - o *2:1 Ratio*

Benefits:
- o Here the entire body works to create stability.
- o Tone is brought to the lower body and a great practice of stability and core strength is used.
- o Work not to over-use the arms but transfer that strength into the core region of the body.

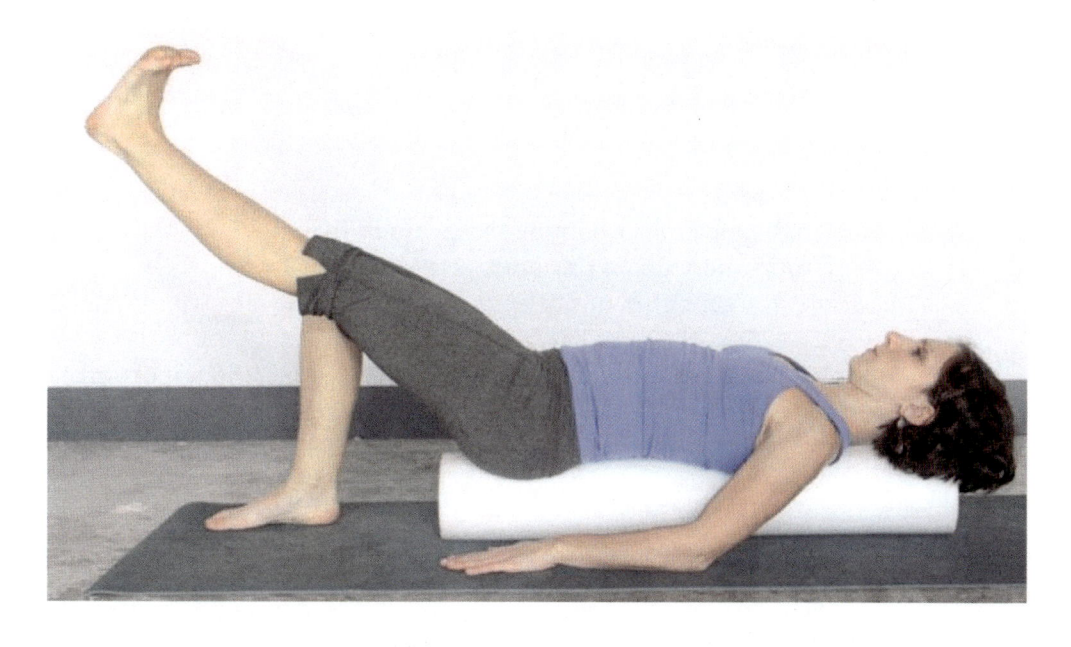

Supine Stabilization Series:
Single Leg Stretch:

To Begin:
- ➢ Lie down onto the foam roller lengthwise in neutral and place your feet on the floor beneath you at hips distance.
- ➢ Choose your supportive arm position.
- ➢ EXHALE; lift the right leg up to ninety-degree angle, followed by the left leg placing the knee over the hip. You can check that by extending a hand towards the knee to touch.
- ➢ INHALE; extend the right leg out to 90° or 45° staying stable on the foam roller (let the stability determine how far to extend) working not to arch the lower back.
- ➢ Keep the extended leg in neutral with the knee pointing upwards towards the ceiling (*not externally rotated*).
- ➢ EXHALE; return the limb back to center hovering above the hips.
- ➢ Be sure not to take the knee further than the hipline and not to sink the spine out of neutral.
- ➢ Repeat the left side in the same manner.
- ➢ Repeat this movement 5 to 10 times and then repeat the opposite side.
  - o *Variations:*
    - *Reach through the ball or the heel of the foot. Or point on extension and flex on return.*
    - *Modified:*
      - *Practice one leg at a time keeping the opposite on the floor and then repeat opposite side.*
    - *Advanced:*
      - *Try this movement with a light hand weights, bend the arms to rest on the elbows (remember to keep palm facing the midline).*
      - *Place a second roller crosswise beneath the foot on the floor.*
  - o *2:1 Ratio*

Benefits:
- o The core is challenged as stability is the primary focus.
- o The legs are tone and worked in neutral.
- o It is important to remember not to externally rotate the legs when extending them not to over-use the hip flexors.
- o Most of us have tight outer hips and glutes already and it is important to the health of our bodies to train neutral first then un-neutral to gain long-term balance and vitality.

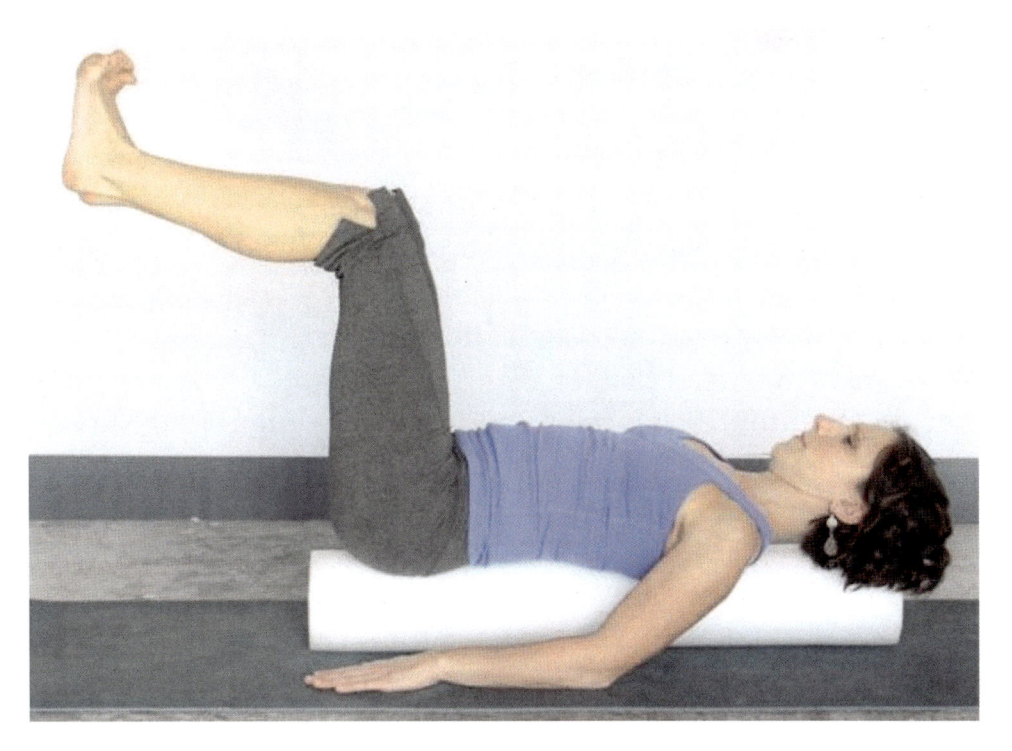

Single Leg Stretch Phase 1: Exhale

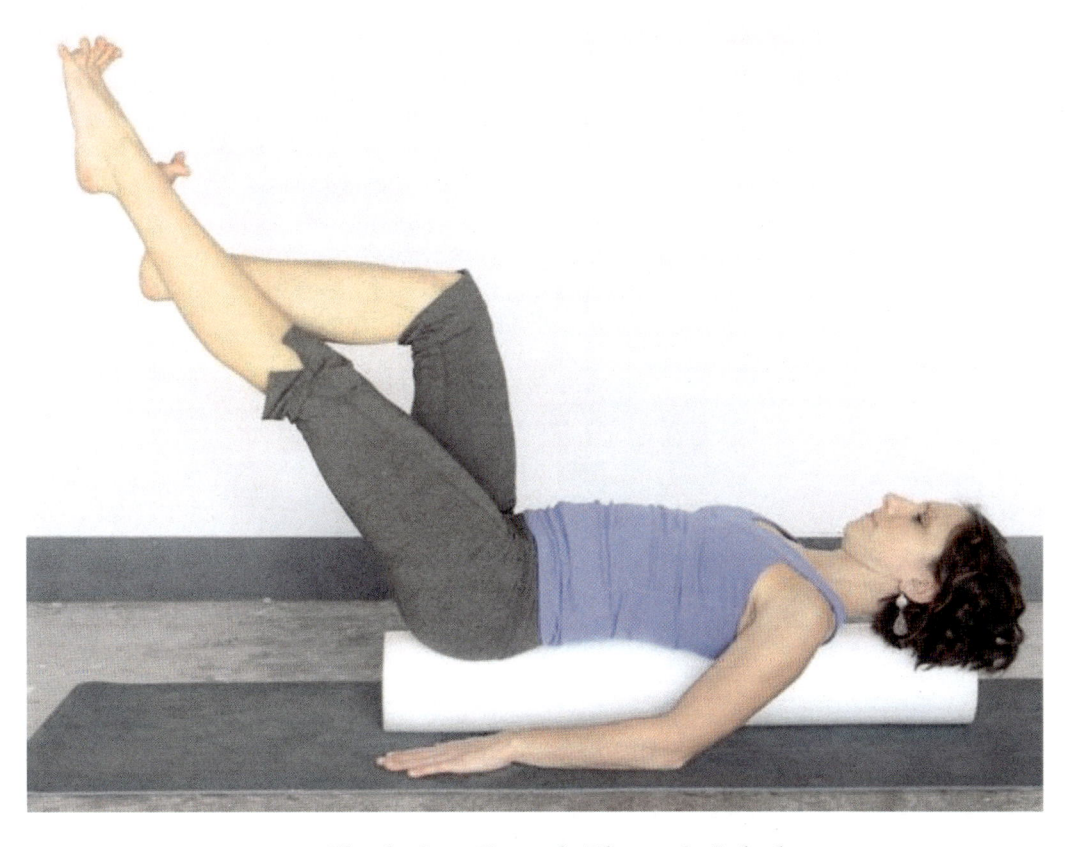

Single Leg Stretch Phase 2: Inhale

Spinal Stabilization Series:
Single Leg and Arm Stretch:

To Begin:
- ➤ Lie down onto the foam roller lengthwise and place your feet on the floor beneath you, at a comfortable distance below the foam roller, at hips distance.
- ➤ Choose your supportive arm position.
- ➤ EXHALE; lift the right leg up to a ninety-degree angle placing the knee over the hip and the left palm in towards the lifted inner knee.
- ➤ INHALE; extend the opposing limbs away from each other, keeping neutral and staying very stable on the foam roller (let the stability determine how far to extend).
- ➤ EXHALE; return the limbs back to center hovering above the body.
- ➤ Be sure not to take the knee further than the hipline and not to move the spine out of neutral.
- ➤ Repeat this movement 5 to 10 times and then repeat the opposite side.
  - o *Variations:*
    - *Advanced:*
      - *Try this movement with a light hand weight (remember to keep palm and inner arm facing the midline).*
      - *Place a second roller crosswise beneath the lower foot.*
  - o *Implement 2:1 Ratio*

Benefits:
- o Balance and coordination are improved and right brain-left brain cross function is at play. Any time we work opposites or cross the mid-line of the body we access both right and left sides of the brain and try to bring them to balance.
- o The body itself is elongated, core and back muscles worked and toned.

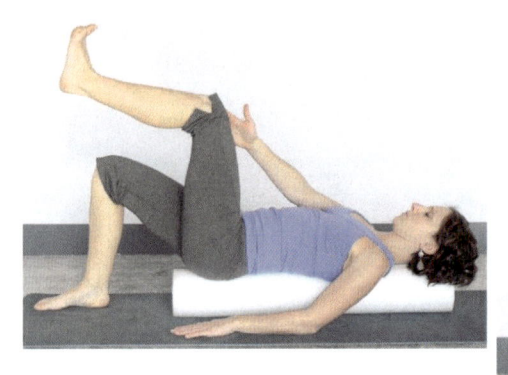

Phase 1: Exhale

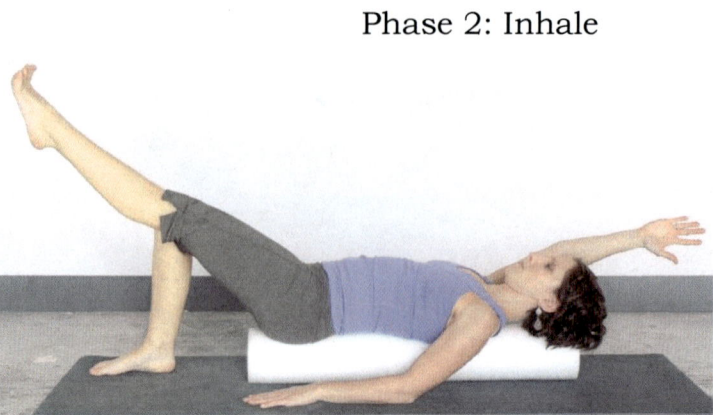

Phase 2: Inhale

Spinal Stabilization Series:
Core Supine Marching:

To Begin:
- ➢ Lying on your foam roller in line with the spine place the feet comfortable beneath the foam roller and find neutral.
- ➢ Choosing supportive arm positions draws awareness to the entire body.
- ➢ Stiffen up the core to gain more support for the body.
- ➢ INHALE, very slowly and mindfully life the right foot only 1-2 inches off the floor (do not go high).
- ➢ EXHALE, set the foot down.
- ➢ Repeat the same thing on the left side, being very careful not to shift on the roller or lose your balance.
- ➢ Continue to march the feet for 30 seconds to 1 minute.
- ➢ Rest and observe how the body feels.
  - o *Variations:*
    - *Try doing this with the arms lifted off the floor.*
    - *Place a small or large acuBall between the knees to bring more mindfulness to the marching and use of the core.*

Benefits:
- o Here you gain stability, body awareness, a sense of core work and mind-body connection.
- o Remember the movement comes from the core not initially from the legs.
- o Keep in mind this is a slow movement so do not rush.

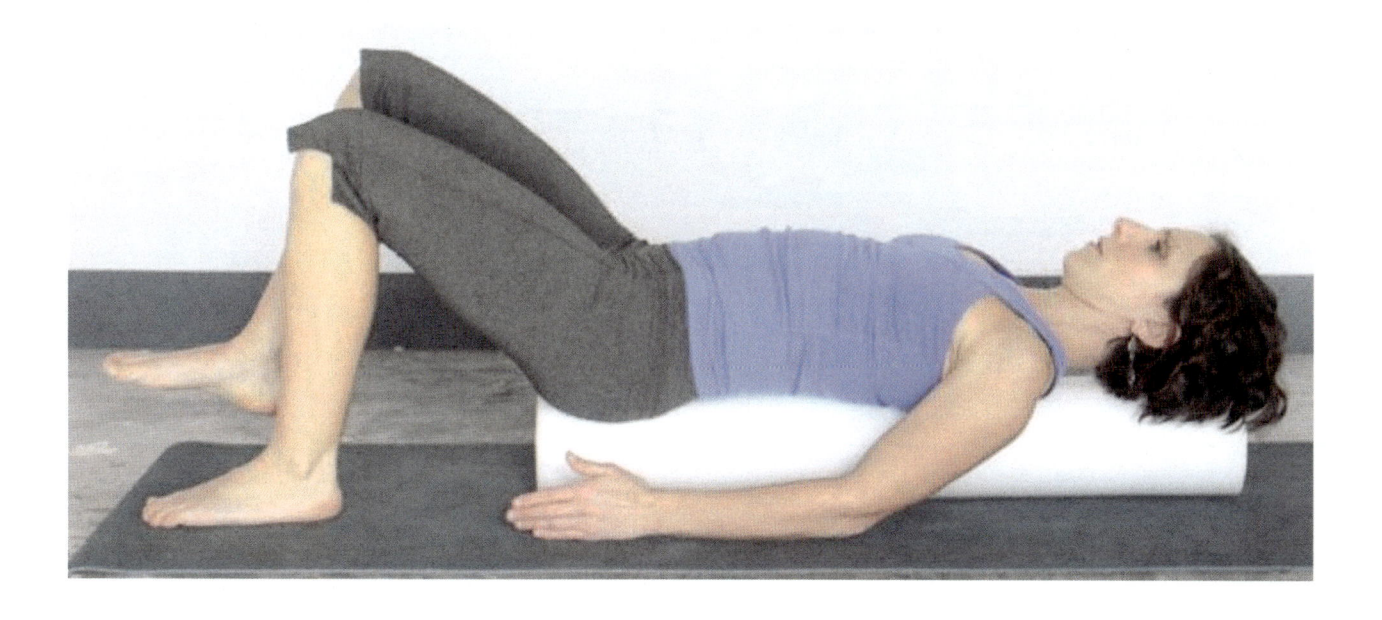

Spinal Stabilization Series:
Articulating Spinal Bridge:

To Begin:
- Lying on the foam roller length-wise, align the head to the tail-bone on the foam roller.
- Choose a supportive arm position and find neutral.
- With the feet at a comfortable distance under the knees at about hips width apart.
- EXHALE, posterior tilt the pelvis and lower lumbar into the foam roller being careful not to over work the gluts.
- INHALE; leading with the tail-bone begin to mindfully roll the spine up off the roller, ending between the shoulder blades (imagine the spine like tape).
- Lift the heels and EXHALE; unroll the spine down into the foam roller one vertebrae at a time back into neutral.
- INHALE, anterior pelvic tilt on foam roller.
- EXHALE, posterior pelvic tilt on foam roller.
- Begin roll up again. Repeat this 5 to 10 times.
    - *Variations:*
        - *Try practicing this with a small ball, yoga block or the large acuBall between your knees to keep the legs hips and core working properly.*

Benefits:
- Here the entire spine, disc and spinal supportive muscles are massaged, the lower back is relieved of tension and the heart is opened.
- This is particularly beneficial for those who suffer from kyphosis (a rounded upper back) and or tight hip flexor.
- Those who sit long term may find relief here.

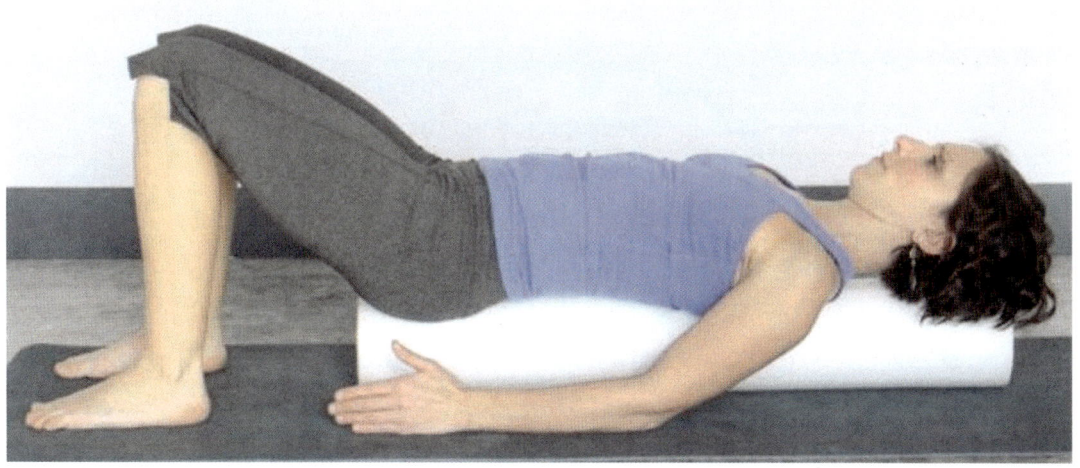

Articulating Bridge Phase 1

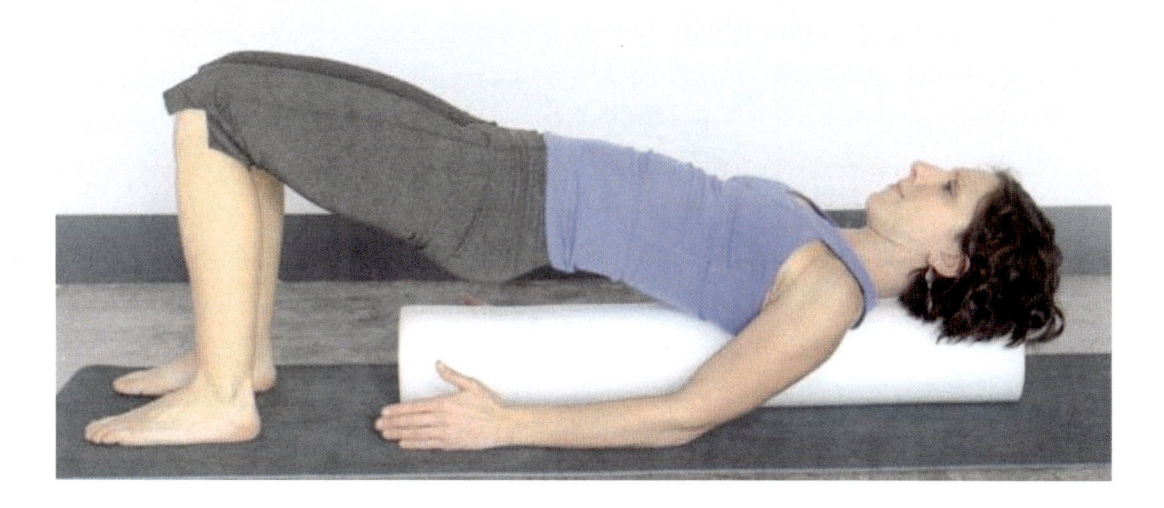

Articulating Bridge Phase 2

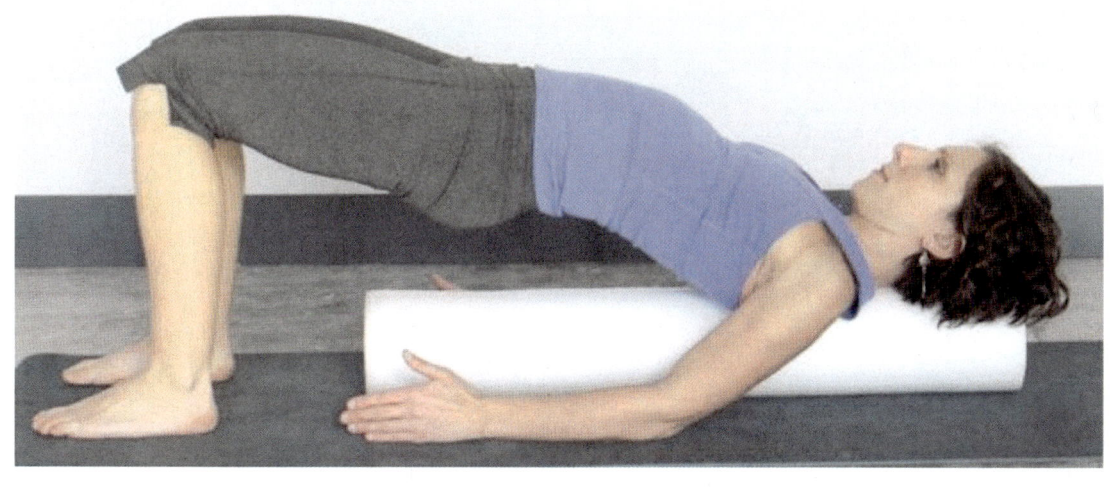

Articulating Bridge Phase 3

Spinal Stabilization Series:
Shoulder Bridge:

To Begin:
- Lying on the foam roller length-wise align head to tail-bone on the foam roller.
- Choose a supportive arm position and find neutral (remember to relax the front ribs down).
- With the feet at a comfortable distance under the knees at about hips width apart.
- INHALE prepares.
- EXHALE, keeping the trunk and spine in neutral, and stable lift the body all at once only as high as you can maintain neutral, not over-use the gluts and breathe calmly.
- Remain here for 3 to 5 breaths, focusing on the exhale to help contract the core.
- EXHALE, return to the foam roller in neutral.
- INHALE, prepare and begin again.
- Repeat this 3 to 8 times.
  - *Variations:*
    - *Place a small ball, the large acuBall or a yoga block between the knees to avoid thrusting the pelvis up.*
    - *Add a second roller under the bottoms of the feet and remain stable.*
    - *Try this with the arms extended vertical to the ceiling.*
      - *Add a protraction/retraction to the bridge:*
        - *INHALE, melt the shoulders back and EXHALE reach the arms up, broadening the upper back. Work not to bend the elbows.*

Benefits:
- Here the spine is worked, hips are strengthened.
- If you know you have tight outer hips and or weak inner thighs use the support between the knees.
- The entire front body is opened and worked while the entire core is active and supportive.

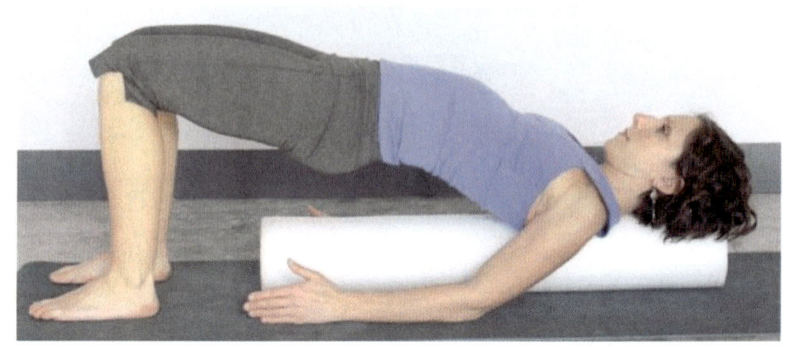

Spinal Stabilization Series:
Shoulder Bridge Variations:

To Begin:
- Lying on the foam roller length-wise align head to tail-bone on the foam roller.
- Choose a supportive arm position and find neutral.
- With the feet hips width apart and the heels beneath the knees place a small ball between the knees.
- Prepare the body and INHALE.
- EXHALE, keeping the trunk and spine in neutral and stable lift the body all at once only as high as you can maintain neutral, not over-use the gluts and keep breathing calmly.
- Remain here and without shifting the body or dropping a hip, imagine a marble in your navel and lift only the left heel off the ground without lifting one leg higher than the other.
- Take 3 to 5 breaths and repeat the opposite side.
- EXHALE; return the torso to the foam roller in neutral.
- Repeat this process 3 times, either moving in and out of Shoulder Bridge or repeat the 3 rounds remaining in bridge the entire time.
    - *Variations:*
        - *Variation 2:*
            - *Move into Shoulder Bridge lift the entire left foot off the floor 1 inch only remain there for 3 to 5 breaths and repeat on the opposite side.*
        - *Variation 3:*
            - *Move into Shoulder Bridge lift the entire left foot and extend the left leg from the knee keeping a straight line from the shoulder girdle to the big toe. Work not to drop a hip or shift with the small ball. Hold here 3 to 5 breaths and repeat the opposite side.*
    - *2:1 Ratio*

Benefits:
- Lower body stability is achieved.
- Tone is brought to the hamstrings and gluteus muscles.
- Stability to the ankles is enhanced.
- Body awareness is gained and balance is brought to both the right and left sides.

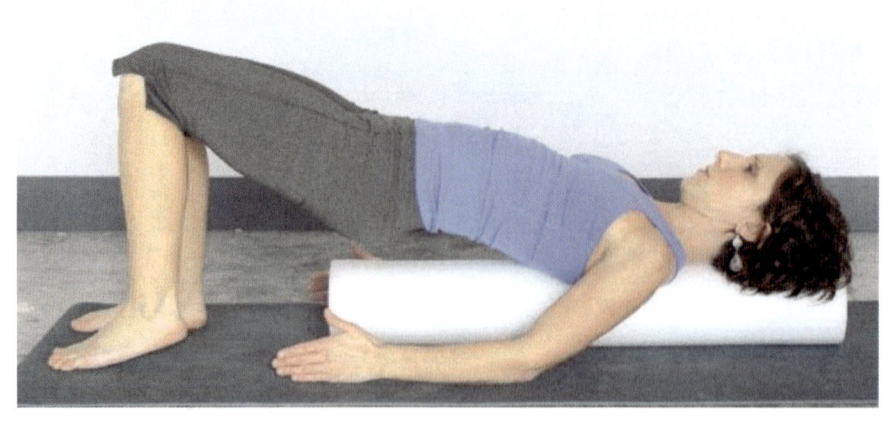

Bridge Phase 1: Heel Lift

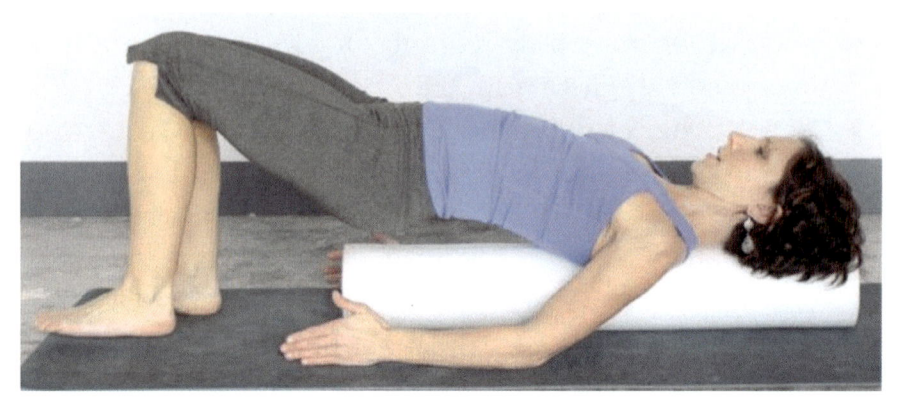

Bridge Phase 2: Foot Lift

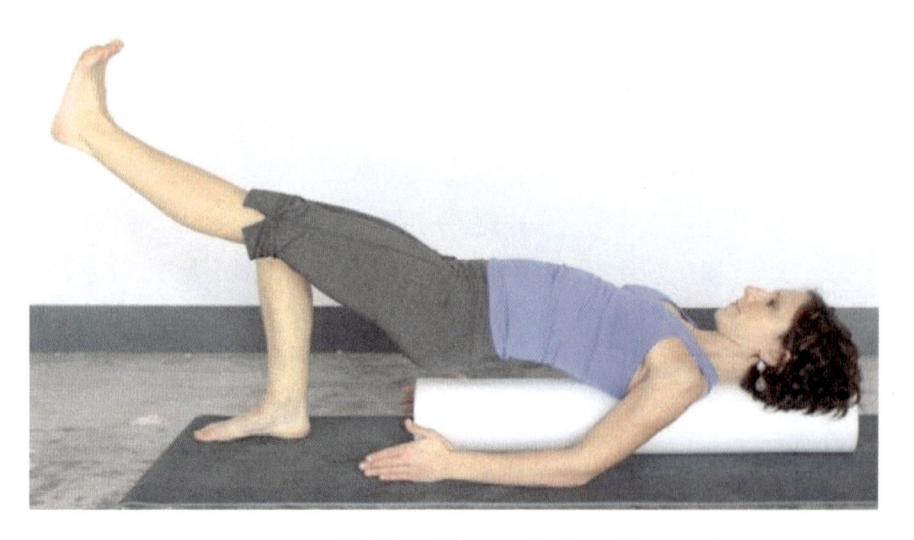

Bridge Phase 3: Leg Extension

Below: Option to place prop between knees for stability.

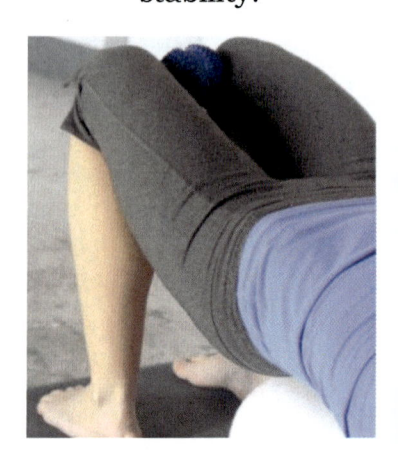

Spinal Stabilization Series:
Leg Circles:

To Begin:
- Lying on the foam roller length-wise align head to tail-bone on the foam roller. With your knees bent and feet at a hips width.
- Choose a supportive arm position and find neutral.
- INHALE; lift the right leg up off the floor to 90°, placing the knee over the hip, and work to keep the lower leg stable and strong.
- Keep the foot flexed and remember to move from the hip.
- EXHALE, firm your core region.
- INHALE circles your leg away from the body drawing a circle the size of a small watermelon to a basketball (here bigger is not better).
- EXHALE to complete the circle.
- Repeat this 3-5 times each direction, noticing stability and try only to move the leg not the rest of the body.
- INHALE to lift the opposite leg to the table top.
- EXHALE releases the right leg down to neutral.
- Repeat this series on the opposite side 3-5 times each direction.
  - *Variations:*
    - *Advanced:*
      - *Fully extend the leg to the ceiling keeping the knee in line with the nose.*
      - *Add a resistance band to the extended foot and hold the ends of the band in the hands.*
      - *Place a second foam roller or small ball under the lower foot either with the knee bent or lower leg fully extended.*
    - *Modified:*
      - *Practice this without the foam roller*
  - *2:1 Ratio*

Benefits:
- This is a wonderful movement to create more mobility and strength in the hip region and deep rotators of the hip if practiced correctly.
- Those with misaligned hips should not practice this movement until hips are realigned.
- The lower core is worked and the quadriceps and hamstrings are both stretched and strengthened.
- This is a great movement to create awareness that less is more.

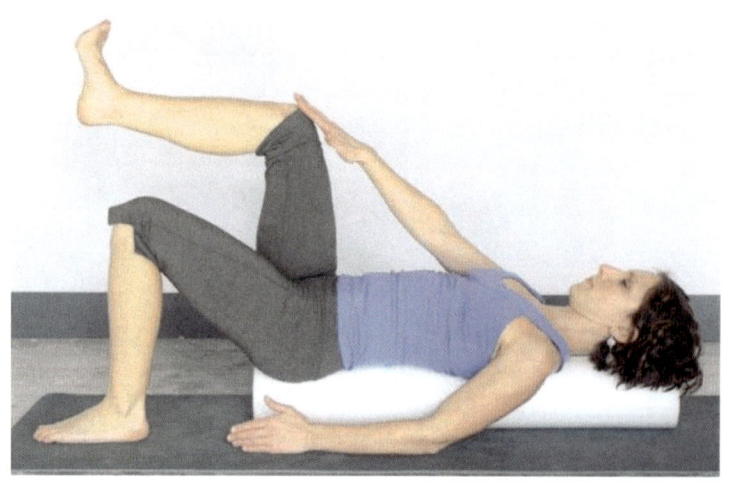

Leg Circles: Modified Variation Phase 1

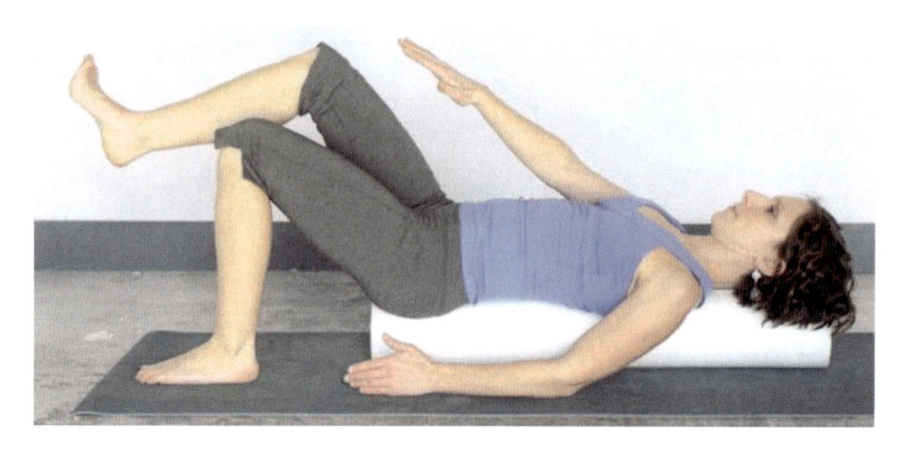

Leg Circles: Modified Variation Phase 2

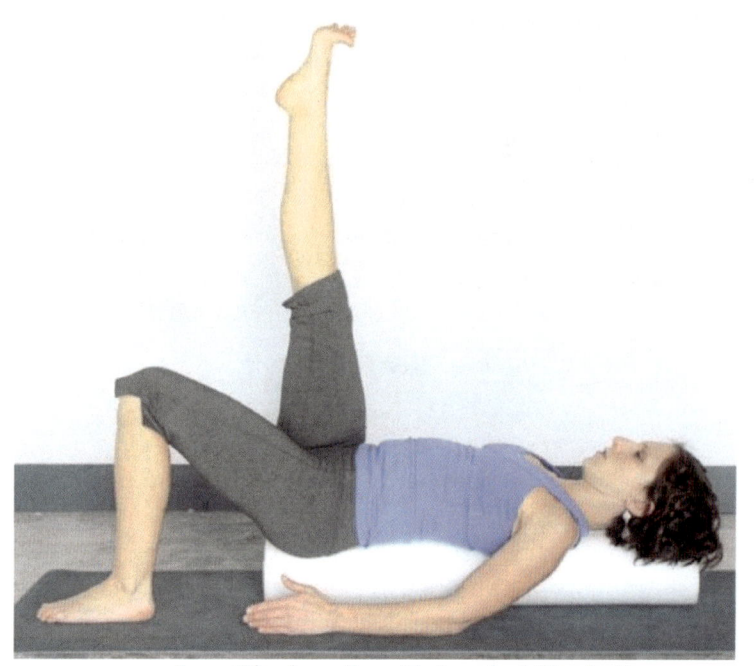

Leg Circles: Leg Extended Variation

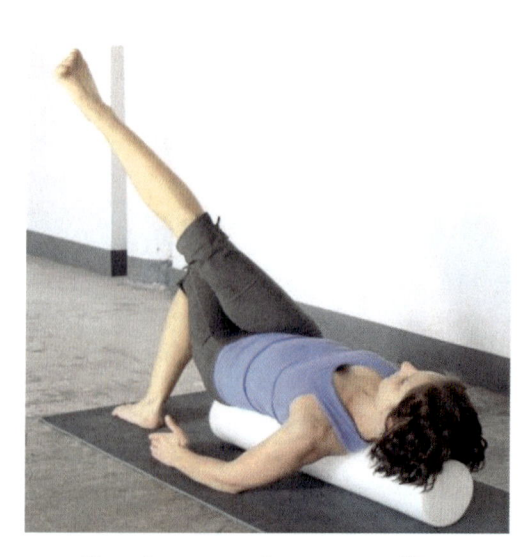

Don't cross the center line of the body

Spinal Stabilization Series:
Foot Push:

To Begin:
- Find neutral and chose your appropriate arm option.
- INHALE and life the legs one at a time to a 90°, table top position.
- Position the feet in a flexed, parallel position with the ankles and knees together.
- EXHALE, extend the legs to a 45° angle.
- INHALE and hold
- EXHALE, return back to starting position.
- INHALE prepare at center.
- EXHALE and begin again.
- Repeat this movement 5-10 times.
  - *Variations:*
    - *Advanced:*
      - *Try INHALING when you extend*
    - *Add a ring between the inner ankles, keeping the legs in a parallel position.*
    - *Add a resistance band around the soles of the feet with the ends held in the hands.*
    - *Modified:*
      - *Only extend the legs to a 90° angle.*

Benefits:
- This movement is usually practiced in an external rotation. However, the majorities of students have tight outer hips and thighs and do not need the extra tightening.
- Remember we want to work and achieve neutral before any other position.
- When practicing neutral the outer thighs and hips are both stretched and strengthened and the inner adductions are made active and equally accessed.
- Mindful core health is achieved.

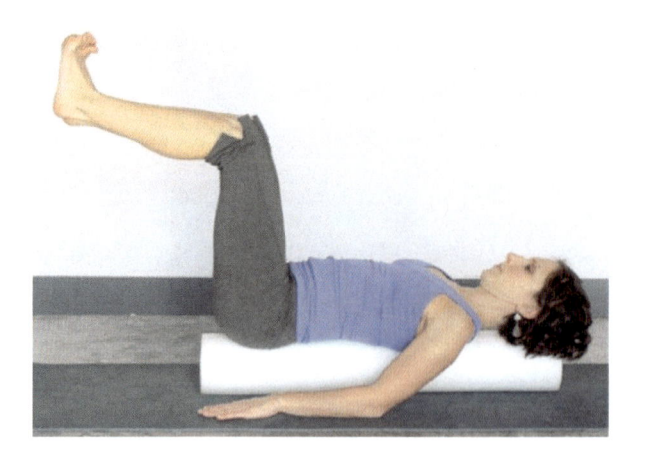

Foot Push: Starting Position

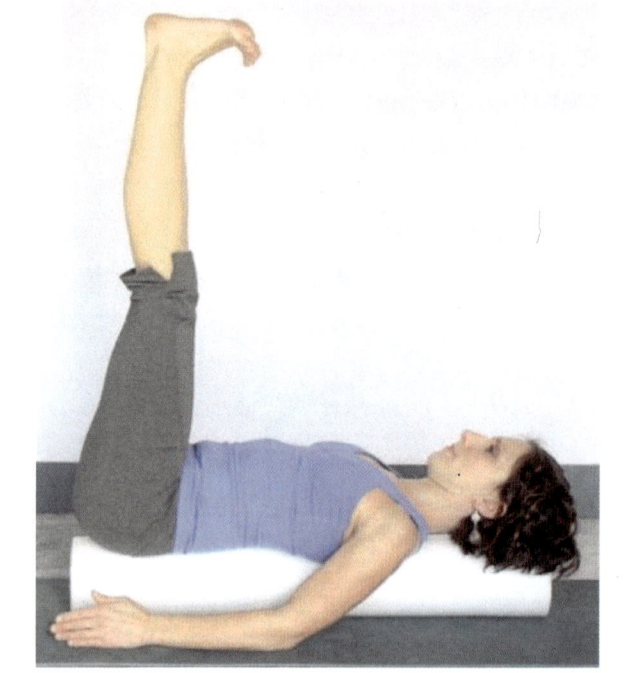

Foot Push: Option 1

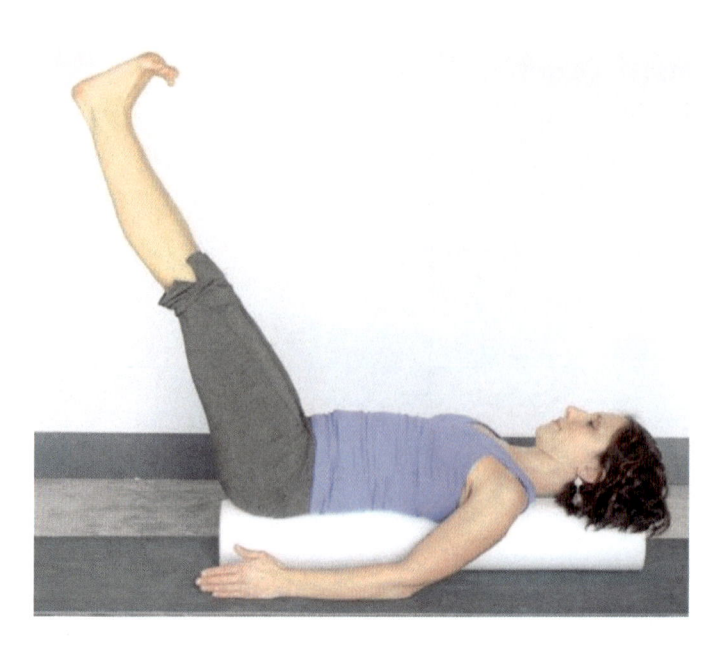

Foot Push: Option 2

Spinal Stabilization Series:
Leg Scissors:

To Begin:
- Lying on your back lift your hips and slide the foam roller underneath your hips and sacrum and your shoulders and head on the floor.
- Resting your hips on the middle of the foam roller find pelvic and spinal neutral.
- EXHALE; lift your legs up to a table top position, knee over hip.
- INHALE and extend the legs fully to a 90° angle, extended to the ceiling.
- Keep neutral with the legs, knees facing your nose.
- Reach actively through the balls of the feet or flex the feet.
- EXHALE; firm your core and in necessary hold the foam roller at each end.
- INHALE; lower the right leg to 45° and draw your left leg towards you.
- EXHALE; draw the legs back to center.
- Repeat this exercise 5 to 12 times.
  - *Variations:*
    - *Modifications:*
      - *Try this exercise with the knees bent; remember to work from the hip.*
      - *Try this exercise on a foam block, or small ball*
    - *Advanced:*
      - *Simultaneously switch legs: INHALE to extend and EXHALE as you switch.*

Benefits:
- This is a great exercise to firm the inner and outer legs and thighs.
- Here we actively work neutral and the muscles that support it.
-
-
-

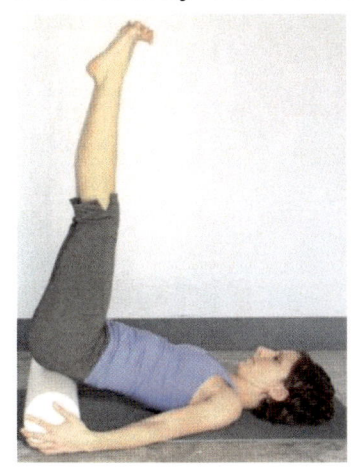

Scissors Phase 1: Exhale   Scissors Phase 2: Inhale

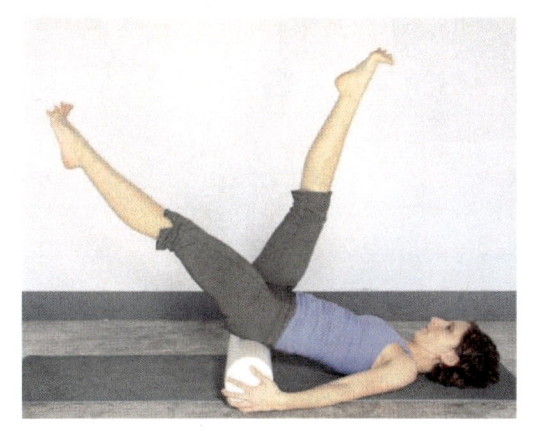

Heel Touch:

To Begin:
- Lying on your back lift your hips and slide the foam roller underneath your hips and sacrum and your shoulders and head on the floor.
- Resting your hips on the middle of the foam roller find pelvic and spinal neutral.
- EXHALE; lift your legs up to a table top position, knee over hip.
- INHALE, lower your right heel towards the floor, keeping the foot flexed.
- Only drop the heel as far as you can remain in neutral.
- EXHALE; float the leg back to the table top.
- Repeat this series 5 to 10 times.
- Repeat this series on the opposite side.
   - *Try this on a small ball or on the floor.*
   - *Experiment extending one leg out to different heights, angles, and rotations as you work to keep your core stable and strong.*
   - *2:1 Ratio*

Benefits:
   - This is a great movement to help work both the lower back muscles, transversus and legs. Be conscious only to go as far as your core and neutral can support you.

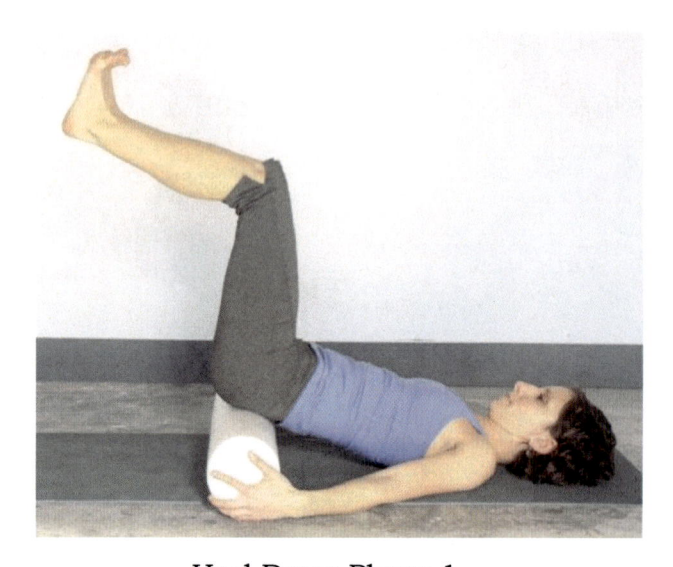

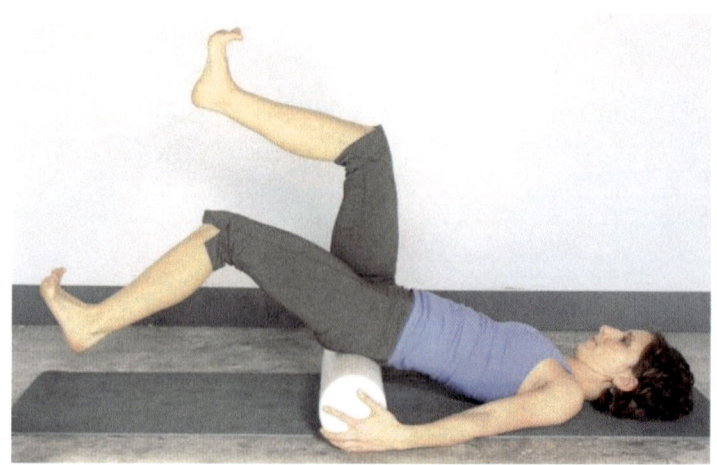

Heel Drop: Phase 1   Heel Drop: Phase 2

Plank Series:
<u>Stretching Cat (aka Swimming)</u>
To Begin:
- Align two foam rollers crosswise on the mat.
- Place the palms on the front roller at shoulders distance and the knees on the second roller hips width.
- Find neutral table.
- Hold here 3 to 5 breaths working to stay stable.
- Keeping stability, slowly INHALE and extend the right leg back placing the ball of the foot on the floor.
- EXHALE; slowly lift the leg no higher than the hip while keeping neutral pelvis and spine (think about the lower belly activating upward as the leg lifts).
- INHALE bend to EXTEND the left arm alongside the ear with the palm and forearm facing inward (think external rotation on the arm).
- Keep the shoulders square with the floor to activate the core even more.
- Hold here 3 to 5 breaths.
- EXHALE; slowly release the limbs one at a time.
- Repeat the opposite side.
- Continue with this series 3 times on each side.
    - *Variations:*
        - *Modifications:*
            - *Extend the arm to "T" rather than by the ear.*
            - *Extend only one limb.*
            - *Keep the back foot down and extend the opposite arm.*
        - *Advanced:*
            - *Extend the limbs simultaneously working hard not to lose alignment of the torso.*
            - *Do not set the back foot to the floor and go directly to an extended position. This is only for those who have good awareness of neutral and can remain there.*
    - *2:1 Ratio (Weaker: Stronger Side)*

Benefits:
- Swimming is a wonderful way to strengthen and create stability in the transversus abdominis.
- This movement helps create elongation in the entire body and tone the legs, glutes, back and arms.
- Working here against gravity is a wonderful way to strengthen the bowl of the abdomen.

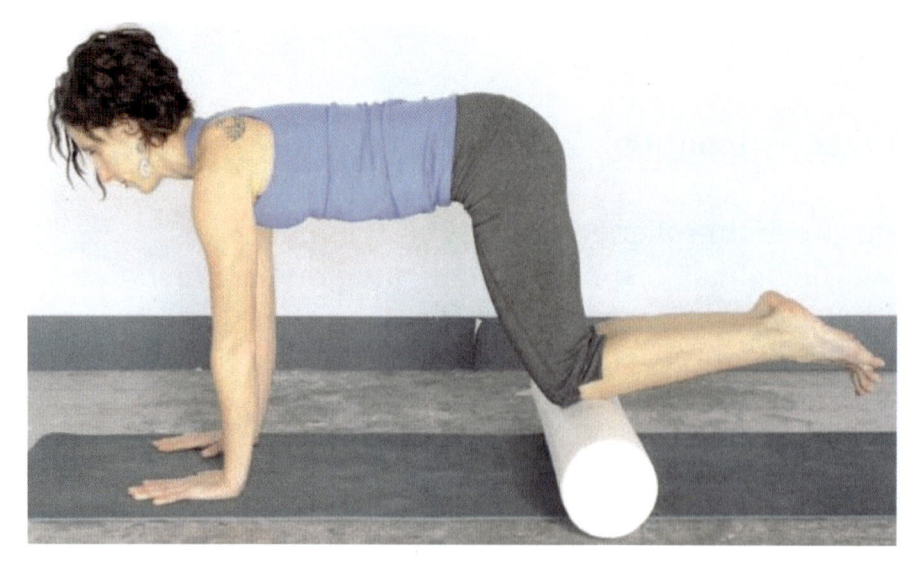

Stretching Cat: Phase 1

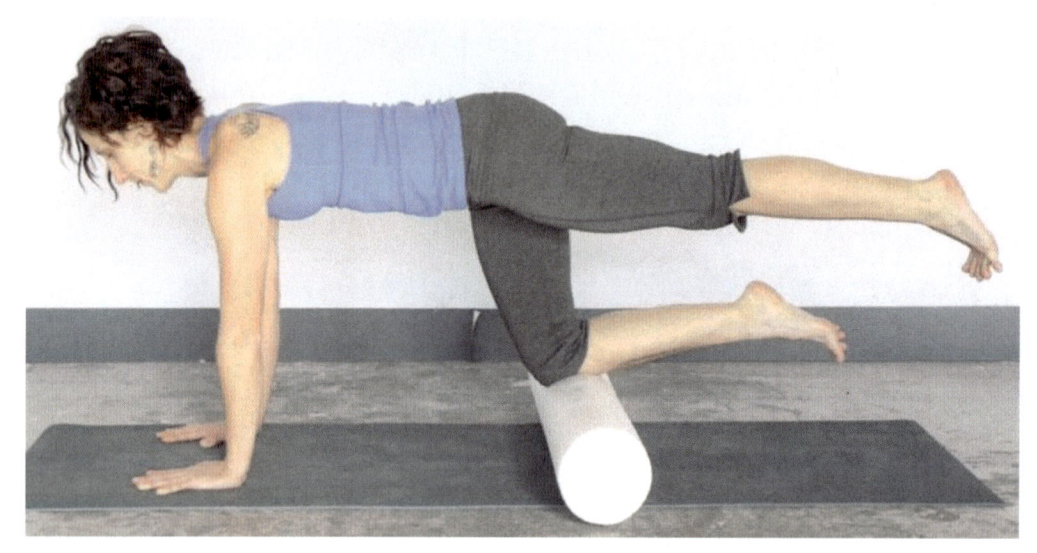

Stretching Cat: Phase 2

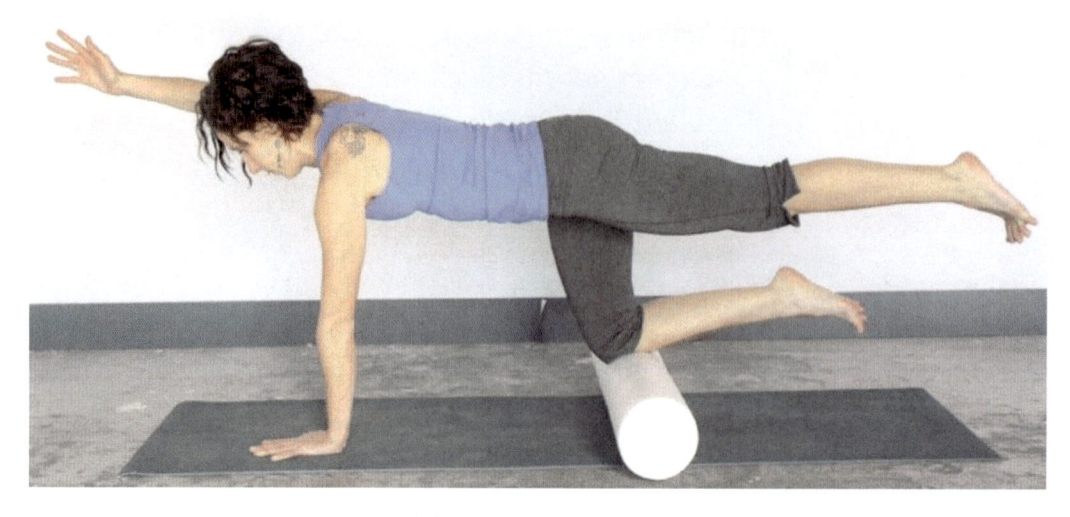

Stretching Cat: Phase 3

Plank Series:
Plank:

To Begin:
- ➤ Place the foam roller crosswise beneath your hands and align your palms and wrists in a comfortable way, shoulder width apart.
- ➤ From a table top position (hands and knees).
- ➤ With the hands on the foam roller align the wrists beneath the shoulders.
- ➤ INHALE slowly and mindfully step the right foot back to a fully lengthened position.
- ➤ Without moving the upper body, EXHALE, step the left foot back to meet the right foot, legs together.
- ➤ Engage the inner thighs and press actively the quadriceps into the hamstrings.
- ➤ Activate the core region of the body by "stiffening" the torso. Press the front hip bones (ASIS) upward and inward towards the deep belly to co-contract the core even more.
- ➤ Press the palms into the foam roller and broaden the back keep the head in neutral not to drop.
- ➤ Hold actively for 5 to 10 breaths.
- ➤ EXHALE lower to the knees and sit to the heels to release.
    - *Variations:*
        - *Modification:*
            - *Once in Plank drop the knees directly down to the floor, placing them behind the hips creating an angle from head to knee.*
            - *Come to the forearms.*
        - *Advanced:*
            - *Come up to the tips of the toes and balance*
            - *Add a second foam roller under the feet and rest on the tops of the feet keeping the ankles aligned.*

Benefits:
- Planking is one of the best ways to work and access the transverses abdominis.
- Here we are working against gravity which is extremely beneficial for the core at all layers.
- When we look at Plank in thirds less stress is on the shoulder girdle and wrists and distributed more evenly through the body.

Plank Series:
Knee Pull: Double:

To Begin:
- ➤ Starting with the roller underneath the shins aligning the roller below the knee.
- ➤ Place the hands under the shoulders.
- ➤ INHALE; extend the legs out checking the roller to be under the knee on the shin, lengthen through the toes.
- ➤ Find a neutral plank.
- ➤ EXHALE firm the core and begin to take the knees inward towards the abdomen, imagining a glass of water on your back not to spill.
- ➤ Watch carefully not to exaggerate the hips lifting to tuck the knees.
- ➤ INHALE, and carefully begin to extend the legs back to a plank-like position.
- ➤ Repeat this series 3 to 8 times, only as many as you can continue to use the core region of the body.
  - o *Variations:*
    - *Try to place a yoga block on your sacrum to test the ability to truly "tuck" the knees underneath your body.*
    - *Pad under the wrists for additional support.*

Benefits:
- o This is a challenging movement and a great one for the transversus abdominis.
- o If the inner core is weak one may feel this more in the hip flexors and should avoid this movement until feeling stronger.
- o Great core based movement for yoga postures like Crow Pose.

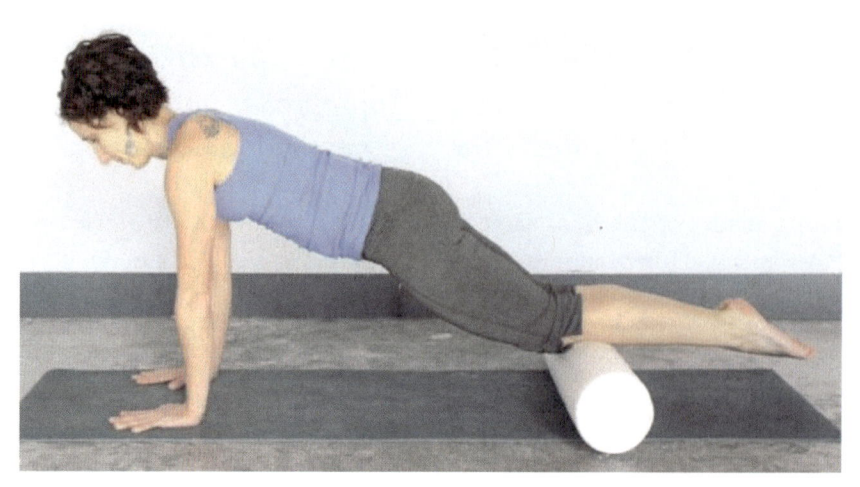

Knee Pull Double: Phase 1

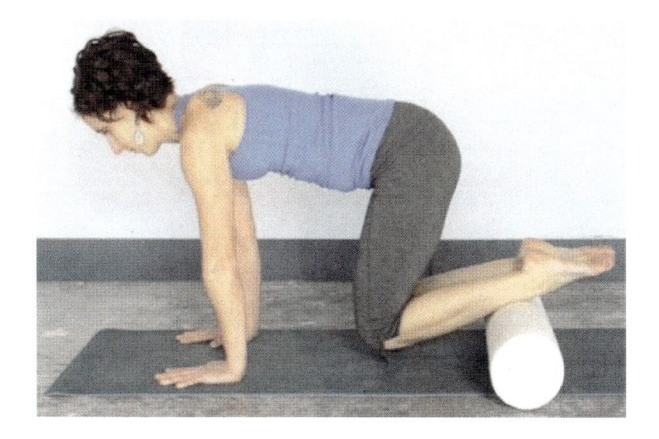

Knee Pull Double: Phase 2

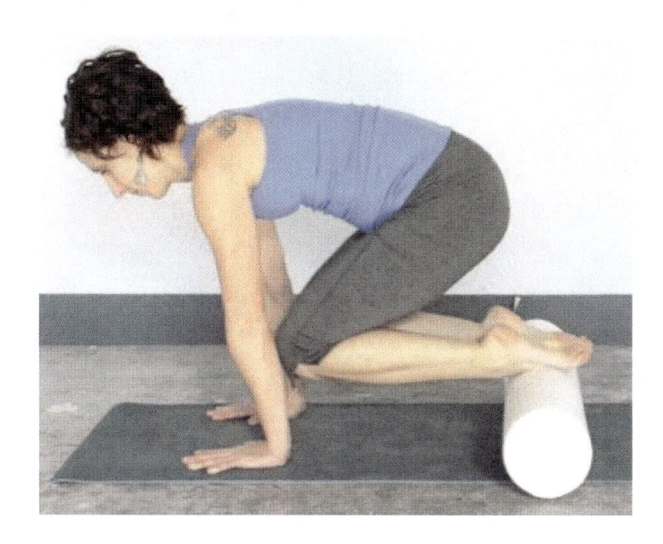

Knee Pull Double: Phase 3

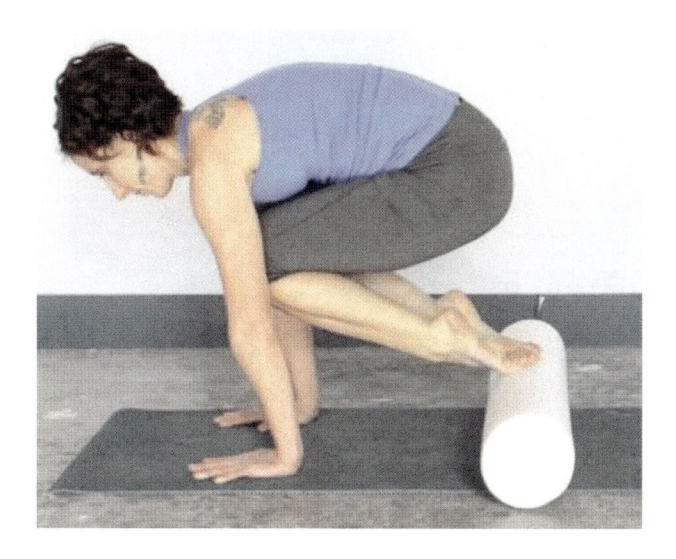

Above: Knee Pull Double: Phase 4

Right: Knee Pull Double: What not to do.

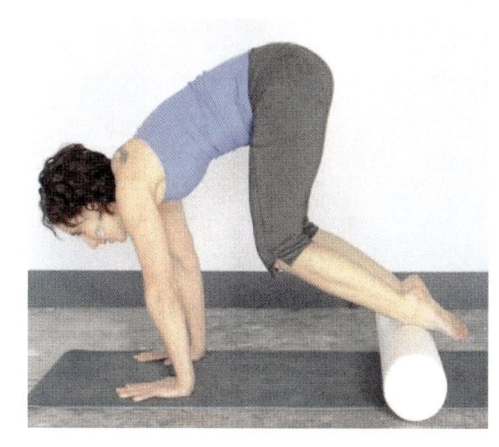

Plank Series:
Knee Pull: Single:

To Begin:
- Start with the foam roller beneath the shins, below the knee.
- Place the hands at shoulders width comfortably on the mat.
- INHALE, extend the legs out to a fully lengthened position, feeling much like a plank.
- EXHALE, pause here and firm the legs, core and press actively into the arms.
- INHALE, lift only the right leg to no higher than hip height (1-4 inches), reaching actively through the foot.
- EXHALE; roll the left leg in underneath the torso into a tucked position.
- INHALE; unroll the leg back to start.
- EXHALE release the right leg back to the foam roller and repeat the opposite side.
- Work each side 1 to 3 times.
  - *Variations:*
    - *Advanced: Continuously work on one side and then repeat the series on the opposite side.*
      - *Modified: Simply lift one leg and just hold, do not tuck the leg.*
  - *2:1 Ratio*

Benefits:
- Single knee pull is a challenging exercise and is not appropriate for those new to the roller or core work.
- This movement challenges the legs, pelvic floor and transversus abdominis.
- The arms and shoulders are worked as they are kept stable.

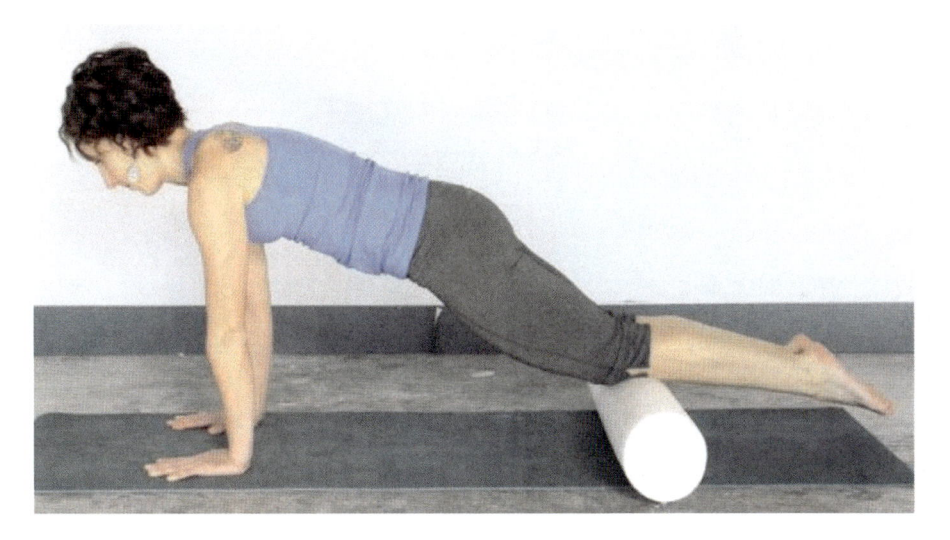

Knee Pull Single: Phase 1

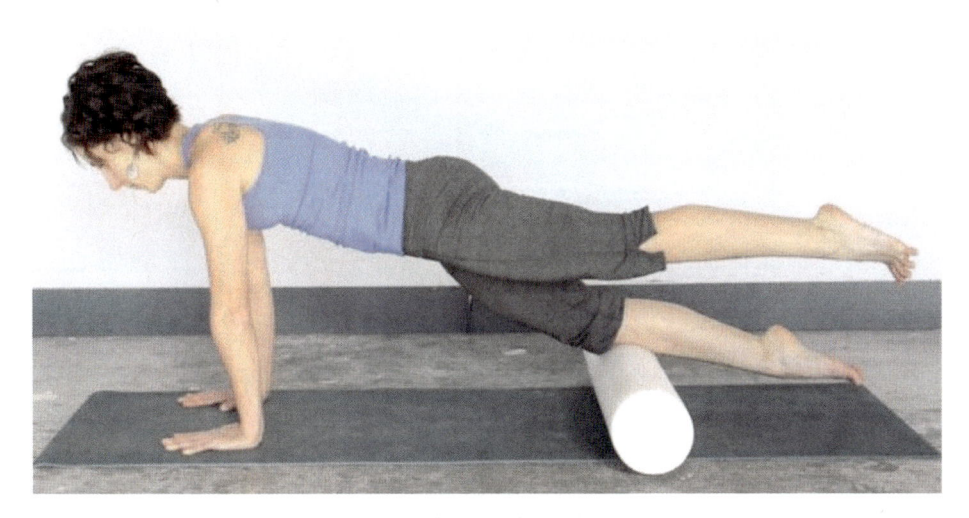

Knee Pull Single: Phase 2

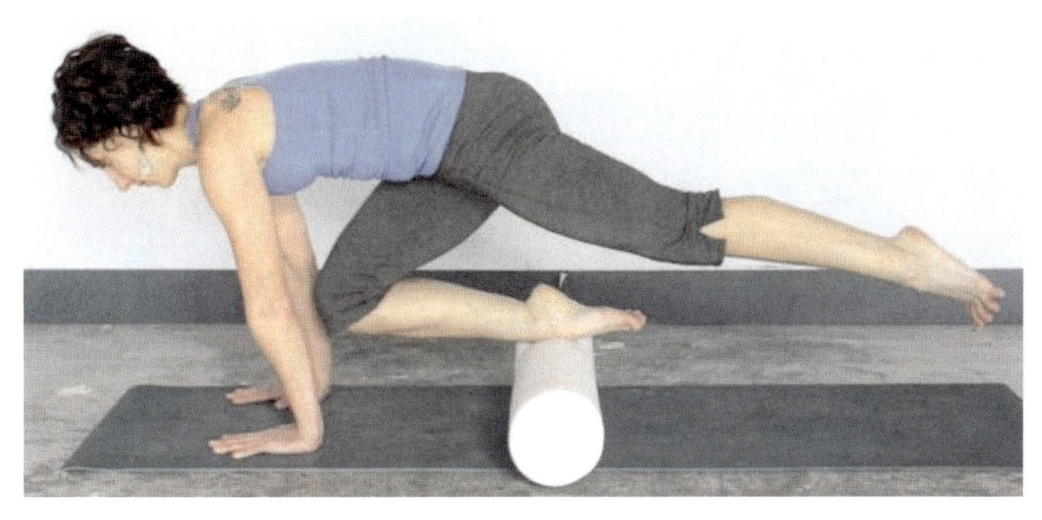

Knee Pull Single: Phase 3

Plank Series:
Pike:
To Begin:

- Find Plank with the foam roller just below the knee on the shins.
- Place the hands under the shoulders with the fingers wide and the eyes of the elbows facing forward.
- Keep the ankles aligned for the entire movement, and firm the thighs into each other.
- INHALE, contracting the deep inner core muscles of the torso, press into the hands and work the hips upward towards the ceiling.
- Pause with the roller near or on the ankles or tops of the feet.
- EXHALE, with control and a firm core, slowly release the body back into a plank-like position being careful not to drop with gravity too quickly.
- Repeat this Pike 3 to 5 times, only repeating as many as you can execute with form and control.
    - Variations:
        - Pad the palms to help with any wrist strain.
        - Try this facing a wall, to pike the hips up and the back into the wall to help with alignment.

Benefits:

- Promotes upper body strength and core stability.
- It effectively works the shoulders, deltoids, and deep inner core muscles.
- The entire back is worked especially as you release back into Plank, working to keep alignment and not fall too quickly.
- If the core is not strong enough, one may easily use the hip flexors to perform this movement.

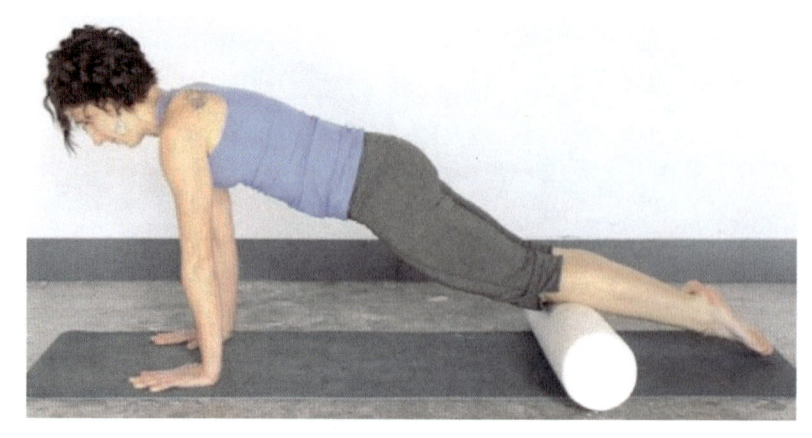

Pike: Phase 1

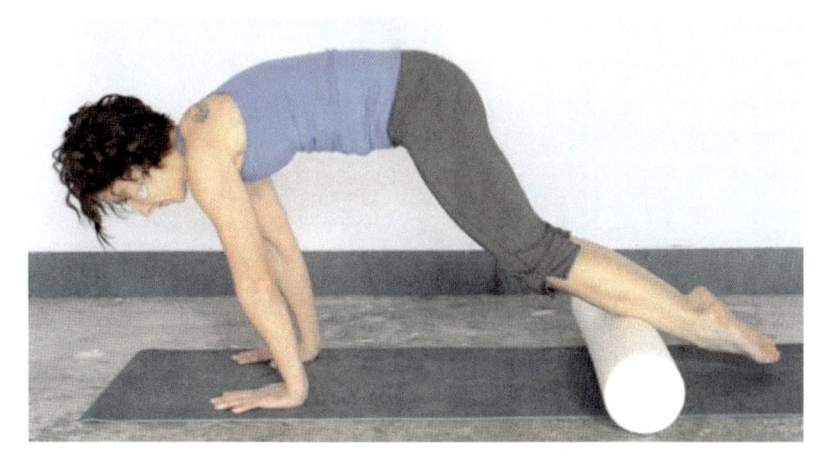

Pike: Phase 2

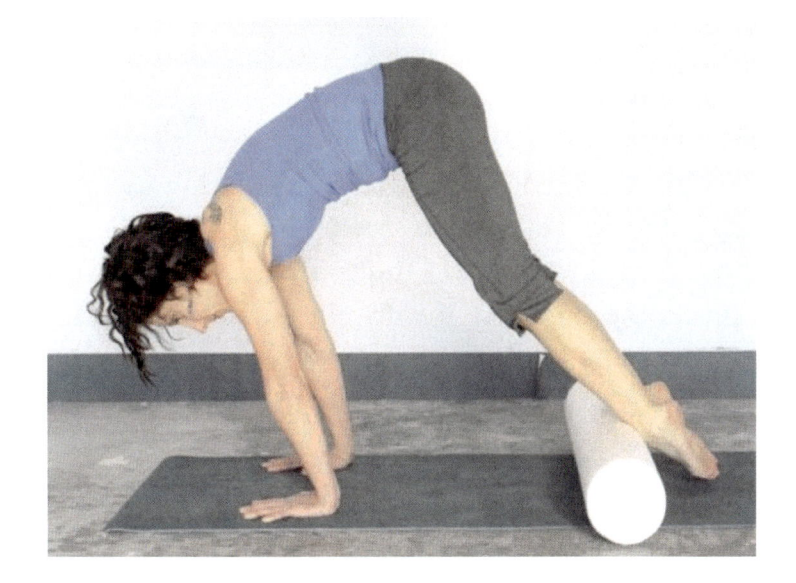

Pike: Phase 3

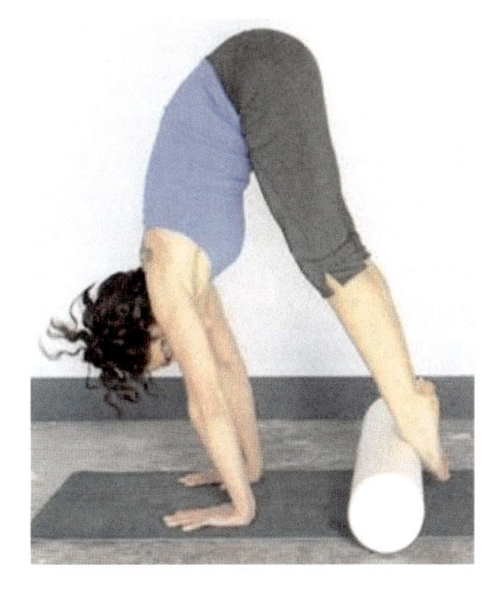

Pike: Phase 4

Plank Series:
Push-Up:

To Begin:
- ➢ Place the foam roller crosswise on the mat and your hands on the roller at shoulders width apart.
- ➢ From your knees, slowly step back the feet one at a time to a Plank position.
- ➢ Align the legs together, and the wrists underneath the shoulders.
- ➢ INHALE, and prepare the body and slightly push with the toes your body forward over the foam roller.
- ➢ EXHALE; begin to bend the elbows to lower the torso down no lower than the elbow being in line with the shoulder.
- ➢ As the body lowers work to keep the core and legs firm, feel as though you are pushing upward as the body moves downward.
- ➢ Allow the roller to move as you lower.
- ➢ INHALE; hold and hover above the mat.
- ➢ EXHALE, press the body back into plank and work the legs and core actively as you press back up.
- ➢ Repeat the Push-Up 3 to 5 times, only as many as you can keep alignment.
    - o *Variations:*
        - *Modifications:*
            - *Practice this on your knees to help keep the body from drooping as you lift and lower.*
            - *Lower in full Push-Up and return back to Plank on the knees.*
        - *Advanced:*
            - *Place a second roller under the ankles, keeping the legs aligned together and strong.*

Benefits:
- o Push-Up is a great movement to work the entire body, but is often thought of only as an upper body movement.
- o Think of the body in thirds: one-third legs strong, one-third core strong and one-third arms and shoulders strong.
- o Here the entire body is worked and challenged for a total all body toner. It is important to practice the variation that you can perform to the best of your ability but yet still be comfortably challenged. This way you continue to use the appropriate muscles for the job.

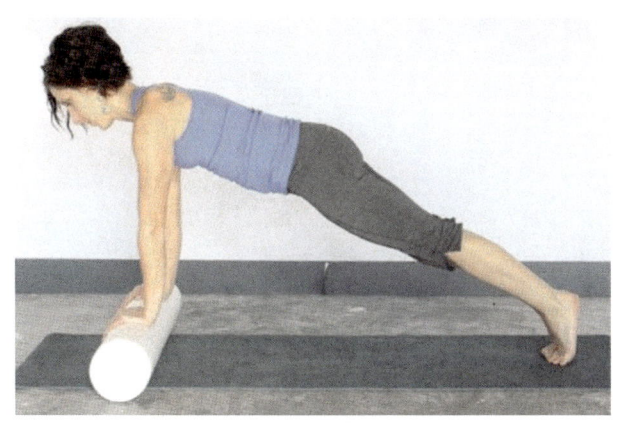

Push Up Phase 1: Inhale

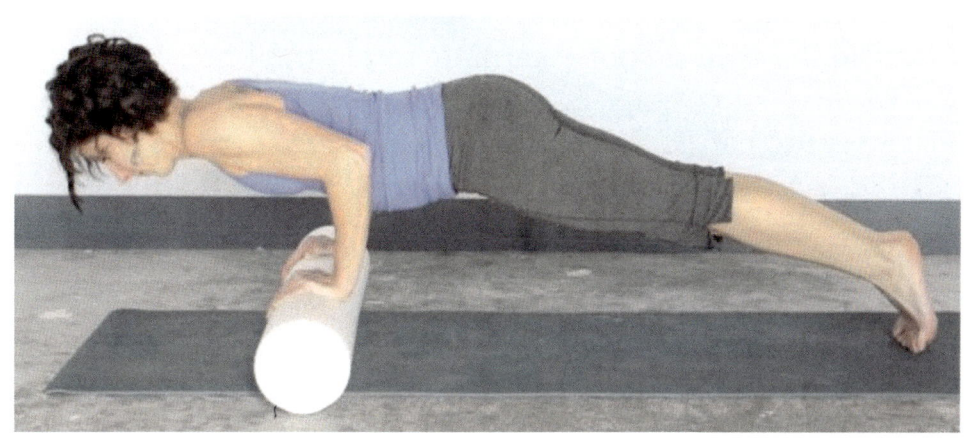

Push Up Phase 2: Exhale

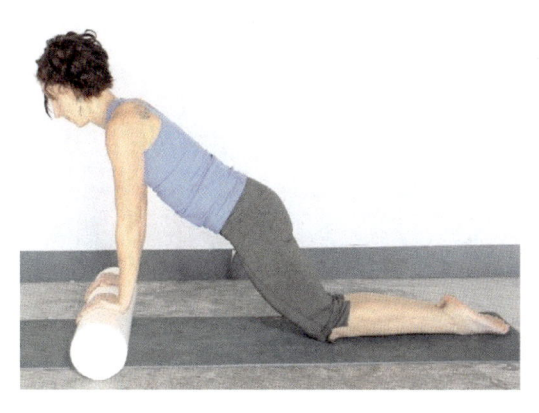

Modified Push Up: Phase 1

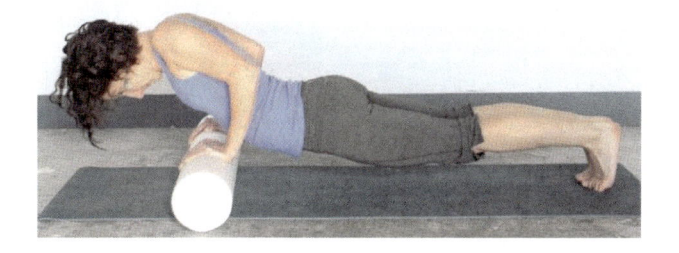

Push Up: What not to do.

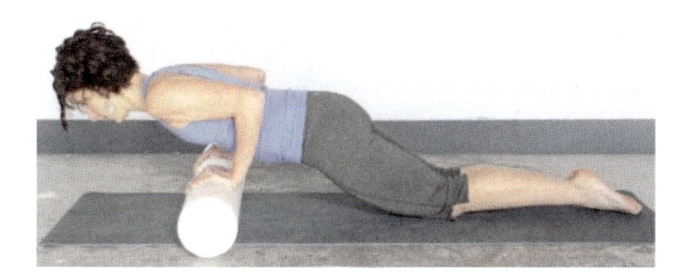

Modified Push UP: Phase 2

Plank Series:
Reverse Plank:

To Begin:
- Place the foam roller crosswise behind you and place the palms on the foam roller fingers pointing towards the body.
- Hug the elbows towards each other, keeping the folds facing your knees, lift from the front chest.
- With the legs extended, activate the inner thighs and press the big toes down into the mat (do not externally rotate the legs).
- INHALE, and lift the hips and legs off the floor, pressing into the foam roller with the hands and arms, allowing the elbows to lengthen last.
- EXHALE; contract the entire body to help maintain support.
- Feel the scapulae pull in towards the spine and slightly downward to help open the chest as you work to keep the chin close to the chest not to collapse the back of the neck.
- Turn the knees upward and try not to rest on the outer edges of the feet.
- Hold here 3 to 5 breaths.
- INHALE return to the floor.
- EXHALE counter pose with a bound angel or forward bend.
    - *Variations:*
        - *Modification:*
            - *Try Reverse Table: knees bent and feet flat to the floor, work to lift the hips to knee and shoulder level.*
            - *Keep the elbows bent to help keep the front chest open.*
        - *Try this with the foam roller underneath the feet and the palms on the mat.*

Benefits:
- This is a great pose to help open the heart and chest, stretch the pectoral, biceps and deltoids. The back body is toned with the help of the core and grounding of the feet.
- Please note externally rotating the legs and feet in this pose will only over work the outer hips and thighs, something in which for most is already tight.

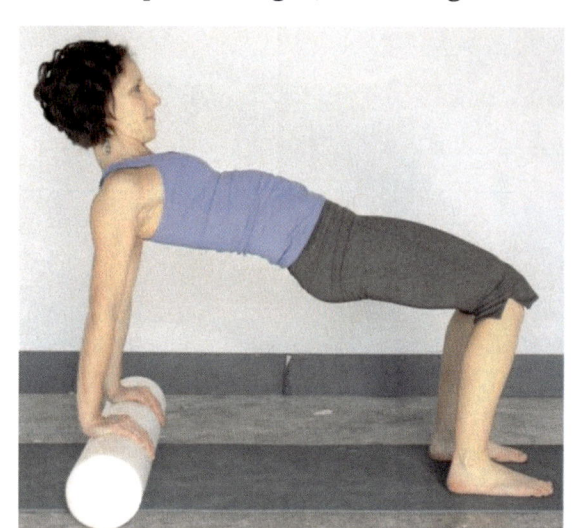

Reverse Table Version

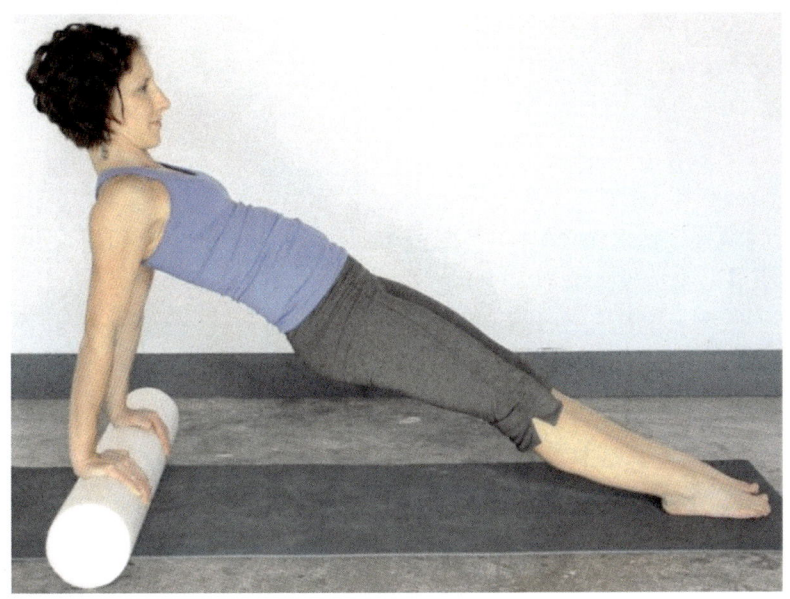

Reverse Plank Phase 1: Inhale

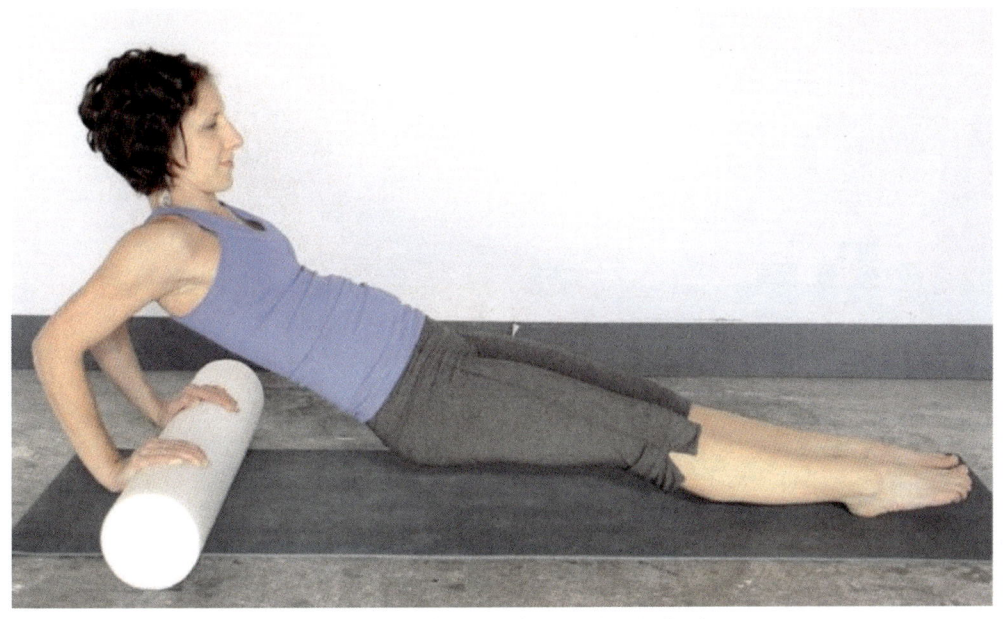

Reverse Plank Phase 2: Exhale

Right: Do not roll to the outer edges of your feet.

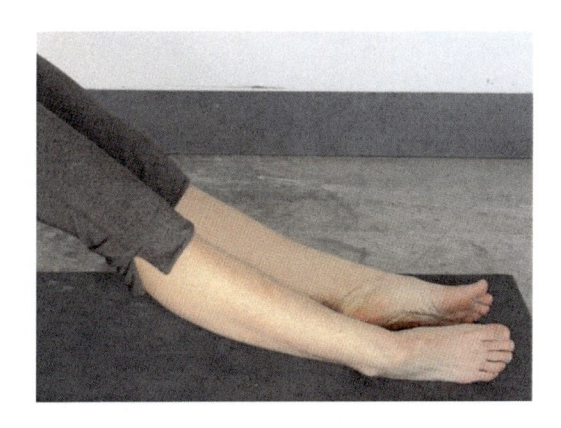

Forearm Plank Series:
Forearm Plank:

To Begin:
- Start on your knees with the foam roller crosswise placing your forearms parallel onto the forearm roller.
- Align elbow under the shoulder and broaden the back without hunching.
- Press down working to keep the wrist and elbow level (remember this for the entire forearm series).
- INHALE; lift the knees up off the floor keeping the legs together.
- Activate the entire body evenly working legs, torso and arms.
- Hold this pose for 5 to 10 breaths.
- EXHALE release and sit back to the heels.
    - *Variations:*
        - *Modified: Drop the knees directly to the floor into Modified Forearm Plank.*
        - *Advanced: Place a second roller under the tops of the feet keeping the ankles parallel.*
        - *Place a block between the palms for more shoulder and core stability.*

Benefits:
- Forearm Plank works the transversus abdominis equally to Plank and this is a great alternative to those with wrist issues.
- The back is strengthened and here you are working against gravity to help permute core health.

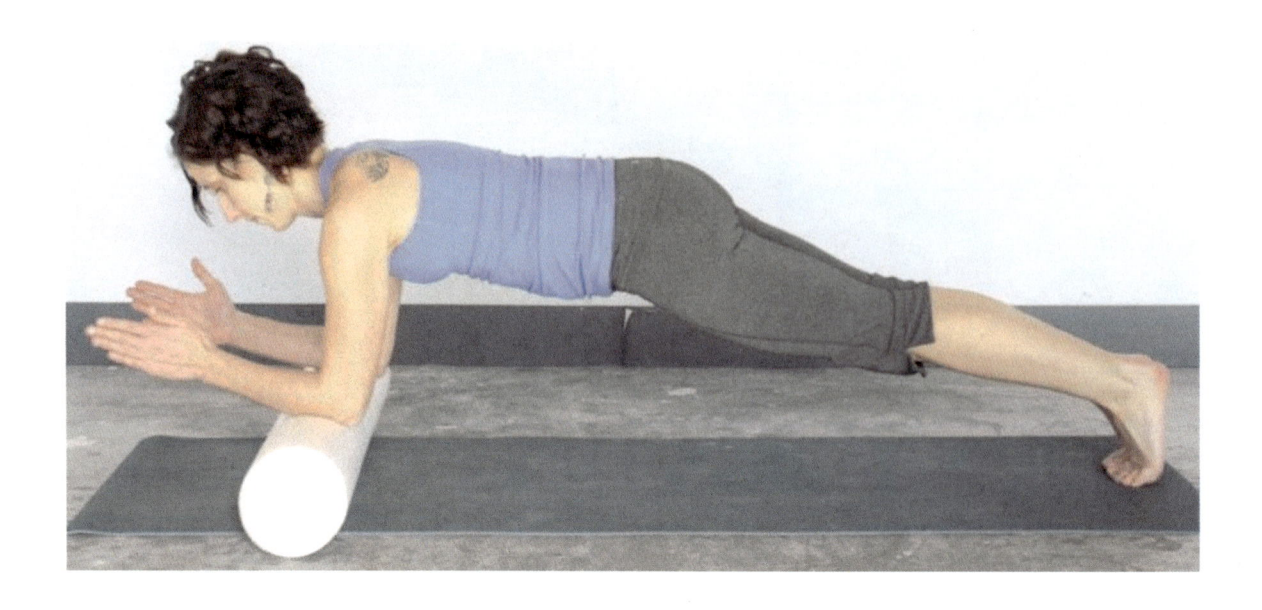

Forearm Plank Series:
Forearm Push & Pull:

To Begin:
- Come to the knees.
- Place the roller crosswise beneath the forearms with the forearms in a parallel position with shoulder over elbow.
- INHALE, step the feet back one at a time into Forearm Plank.
- Align the body from crown to heels in a nice neutral line.
- EXHALE, find Forearm Plank.
- INHALE; roll the forearms out away from the body 2-6 inches.
- EXHALE; return the elbows back underneath the shoulders.
- Repeat this 3-10 times.
- Work not to drop the body and create strain on the back or neck.
  - *Variations:*
    - *Modified: Come to the knees in Modified Forearm Plank*
    - *Place a block between the palms for more shoulder and core stability.*

Benefits:
- Push and Pull helps challenge the transversus abdominis, rectus abdominis, back and shoulder muscles and body awareness. This is not a movement for those with rotator cuff injuries.

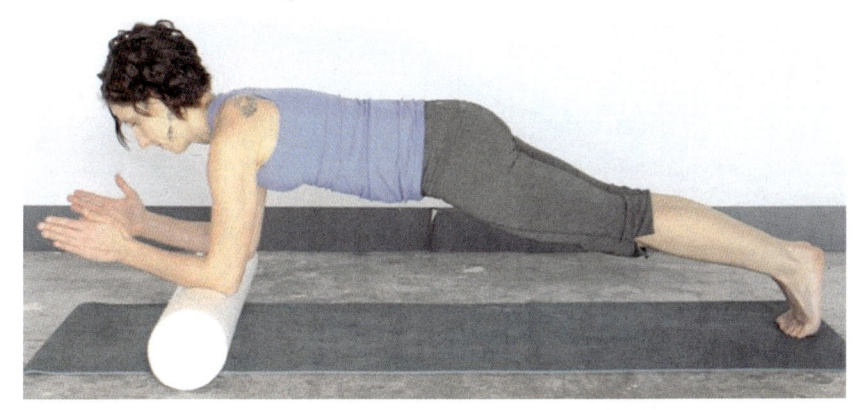

Forearm Push & Pull Phase 1: Exhale

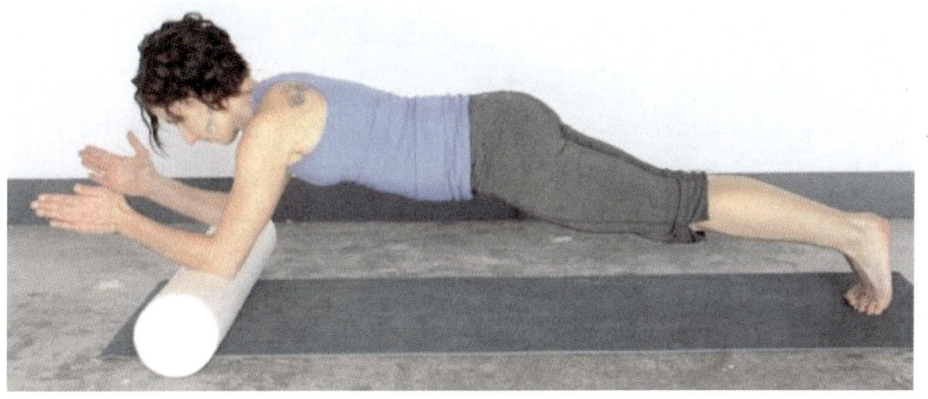

Forearm Plank Push & Pull Phase 2: Inhale

Forearm Plank Series:
Forearm Plank Hip Twist:

To Begin:
- Start on your knees with the foam roller crosswise placing your forearms parallel onto the foam roller.
- Align elbow under the shoulder and broaden the back without hunching.
- From the knees, INHALE, lift the knees into a fully lengthened position and place the feet hips width apart.
- EXHALE and activate the entire body.
- INHALE from the waist twist the lower body only, to the right.
- Putting heel to toe.
- EXHALE and hold, remain here for 3 to 5 more breaths.
- INHALE return to center.
- EXHALE rest back to the heels for a few breaths.
- Return to Forearm Plank and repeat opposite side.
  - *Variations:*
    - *Modifications: When twisting the feet to the right and lower the left knee to the floor.*
    - *Advanced: When twisting to the right anchoring the left foot, lift the right leg to hip height.*
    - *Place a block between the palms for more shoulder and core stability.*
  - *2:1 Ratio*

Benefits:
- This movement is great work for the waist line and oblique's.
- The shoulders are challenged and hips are worked especially in the leg lift option.

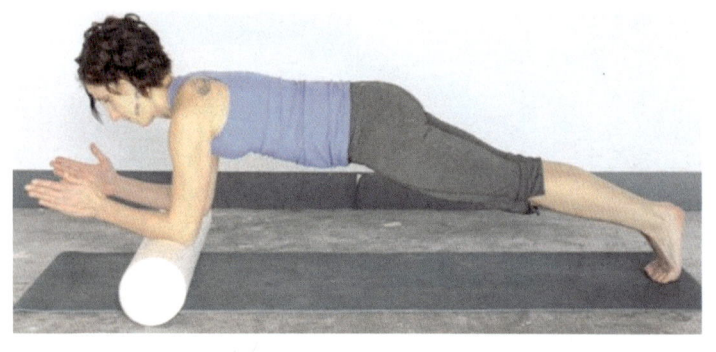

Forearm Plank Hip Twist Phase 1: Inhale

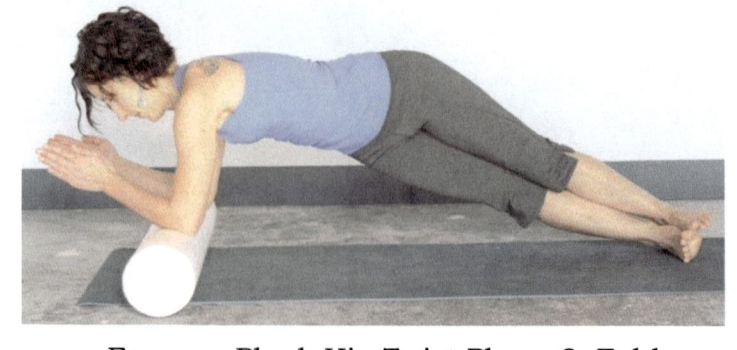

Forearm Plank Hip Twist Phase 2: Exhlae

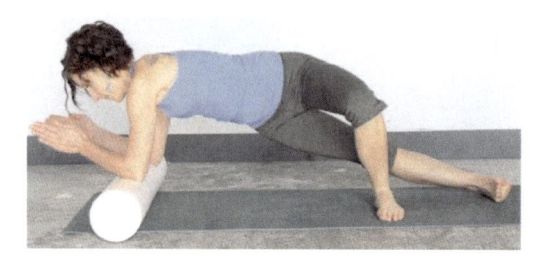

Forearm Plank Hip Twist: Modification

Side Series:
Side Plank:

To Begin:
- ➢ Place the roller crosswise on your right side and lower your right arm at the middle of roller perpendicular to the roller.
- ➢ Resting on your right hip stack or stagger or stack your feet.
- ➢ EXHALE; begin to press the body up off the resting hip to balance on the foam roller and feet.
- ➢ Work to bring the body into alignment keeping the right side body strong and active.
- ➢ Continue to press the bottom forearm down towards the floor to assist yourself from collapsing.
- ➢ Hold here for 3 to 5 breaths.
- ➢ INHALE, lower down.
- ➢ EXHALE, sit back to the heels and rest a few breaths.
- ➢ Repeat the opposite side.
  - o *Variations:*
    - ▪ *Modification:*
      - *Try this with the foam roller underneath the hip and the forearm on the floor.*
      - *Do not use a roller if there is strain or it becomes too difficult to perform safely.*
      - *Place the top legs foot flat to the floor in front of the lower knee for more support.*
  - o *Honor the 2:1 ratio (work the weaker side twice)*

Benefits:
    Side Planking is a wonderful way to get the obliques, gluts, outer thighs and transverses of the core working and active. Side Plank on the foam roller really challenges the muscles of the shoulder and upper back and should not be performed if there is a shoulder injury present.

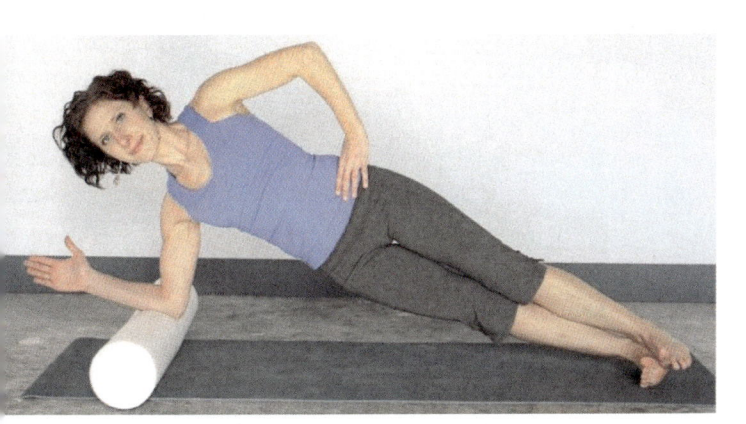

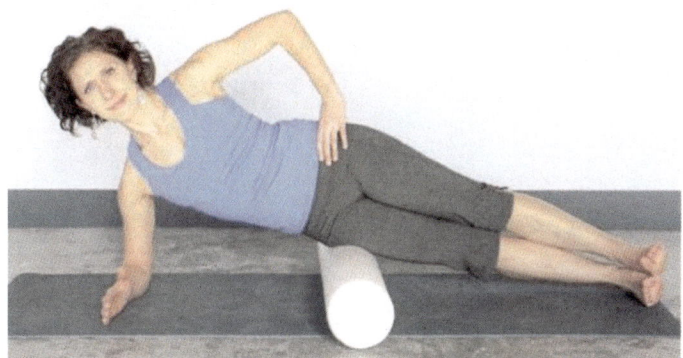

Side Series:
Side Kicks: Up and Down

To Begin:
- Place the foam roller crosswise beneath the right hip, just below the bony protrusion.
- Stack the feet left on right, placing the right forearm on the floor running parallel with the foam roller.
- Activate the lower oblique and lift the lower rib up into the torso to find neutral from heels to crown.
- Draw the legs and feel parallel with each other, working not to lose neutral of the legs as well.
- INHALE, lift the top leg only as high as you can maintain neutral in the torso and lift without externally rotating the hip or thigh (this will not be that high).
- EXHALE return to center, working the core region of the body even more and activating the pelvic floor as you return.
- Repeat this series 5 to 12 times.
- Repeat this series on the opposite side.
  - *Variations:*
    - *Pad the lower elbow if discomfort arises.*
    - *Practice without the foam roller and place a small ball under the oblique for support to practice on the floor.*
  - *2:1 Ratio*

Benefits:
- By strengthening our side bodies, we are able to decrease shoulder and hip concerns.
- Stronger and more balanced hips, glutes and thighs allow us to find more stability when we walk and run. It is important not to externally rotate the leg while moving to help better tone the iliotibial (IT) band, tensor fascia lata (TFL), and not over work the muscles of the inner groin.
- It is important to work neutral, to help create the best strength and stretch combination.
- In the entire side leg series work to keep the hips stacked when working the leg exercises or you will lose the outer hip, glute and oblique work as it is designed.

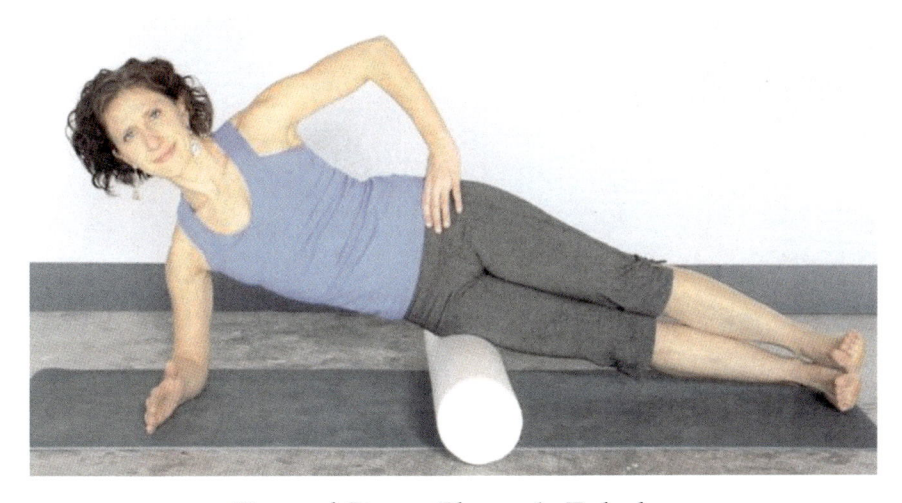

Up and Down Phase 1: Exhale

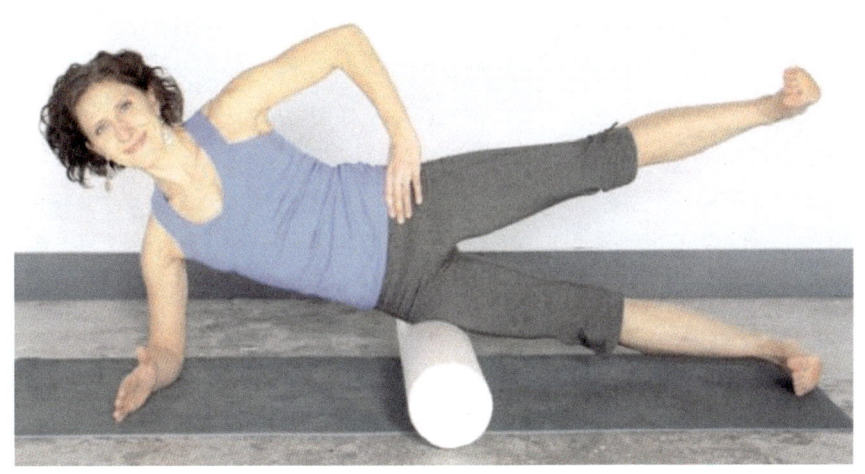

Up and Down Phase 2: Inhale

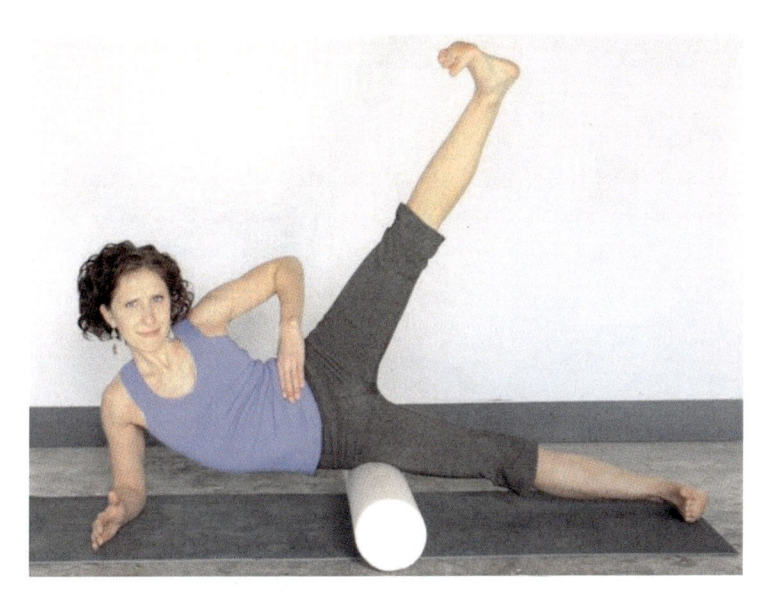

Up and Down: Do not externally rotate the hip and leg

Side Series:
Side Kicks: Front and Back

To Begin:
- ➢ Place the foam roller crosswise beneath the right hip, just below the bony protrusion.
- ➢ Stack the feet left on right, placing the right forearm on the floor running parallel with the foam roller.
- ➢ Lift the lower ribs to activate the lower obliques finding neutral from heels to crown.
- ➢ Draw the legs and feel parallel with each other, working not to lose neutral of the legs as well.
- ➢ INHALE, lift the top leg only as high as you can maintain neutral in the torso and lift without externally rotating the hip or thigh (this will not be that high).
- ➢ EXHALE, pause and recheck neutral.
- ➢ INHALE, move the top leg only as far forward as you body can remain stable, working not to externally rotate the moving leg (imagine kicking the ceiling with the outside of your upper heel).
- ➢ EXHALE, return to center focusing on keeping the lower oblique strong.
- ➢ Repeat this series on this side 5 to 12 times.
- ➢ Repeat this series on the opposite side.
  - o *Variations:*
    - *Pad the lower elbow if discomfort arises.*
    - *Practice without the foam roller and place a small ball under the oblique for support to practice on the floor.*
  - o *2:1 Ratio*

Benefits:
- o Here the hips are toned as in Up and Down.
- o It is important to continue to think of the legs as extensions of the core not to over-use the hip flexors to move the leg forward and back.
- o If there is groin pain, stop the movement or try to lessen the size of the movement.

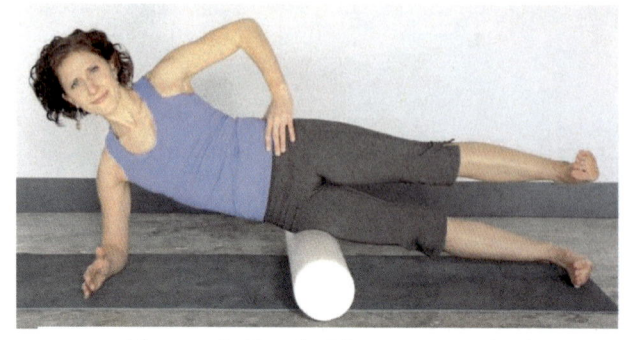

Front & Back Phase 1: Exhale

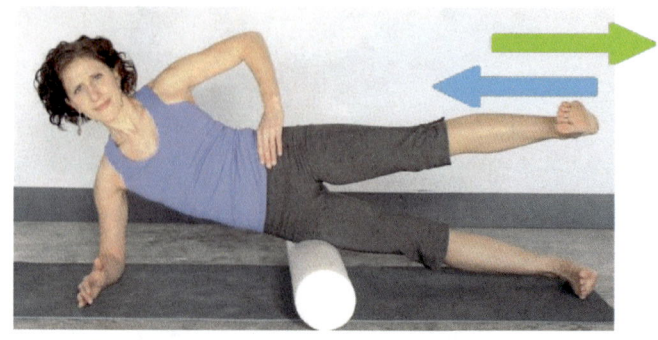

Front & Back Phase 2: Inhale

Side Series:
Side Kicks: Circles

To Begin:
- Place the foam roller crosswise beneath the right hip, just below the bony protrusion.
- Stack the feet left on right, placing the right forearm on the floor running parallel with the foam roller.
- Lift the lower ribs to activate the lower obliques finding neutral from heels to crown.
- Draw the legs and feel parallel with each other, working not to lose neutral of the legs as well.
- INHALE, lift the top leg only as high as you can maintain neutral in the torso and lift without externally rotating the hip or thigh (this will not be that high).
- EXHALE, pause and recheck neutral.
- INHALE circle forward half way.
- EXHALE to finish the circle back to center.
- As you perform the circle, be conscious to keep the body stable, this is a movement in your hip socket not with your entire torso or at your ankle.
- Repeat this circle 3 to 5 times forward and then reverse the circle, 3 to 5 times backwards.
- Release the leg and repeat the opposite side.
    - *Variations:*
        - *Reach through the ball of the moving foot when you circle.*
        - *Pad the lower elbow if discomfort arises.*
        - *Practice without the foam roller and place a small ball under the oblique for support to practice on the floor.*
        - *Advanced:*
            - *Try a larger circle only when you can master the smaller circles, while keeping the body stable.*
    - *2:1 Ratio*

Benefits:
- Here, the hips are toned as with the other Side Series exercises.
- It is important to continue to think of the legs as extensions of the core not to over-use the hip flexors to move the leg forward and back.
- If there is groin pain, stop the movement or try to lessen the size of the movement.
- Circles add movement to the deep rotators of the hips which is important to prevent arthritis and strengthen the hips themselves.

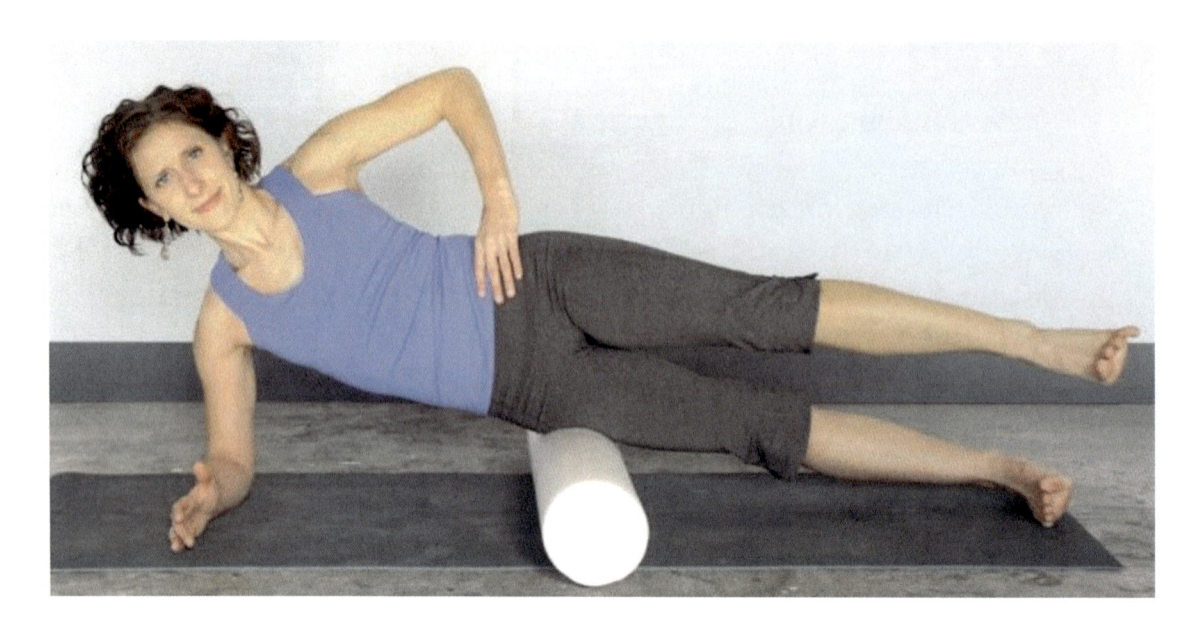

Circles: Phase 1

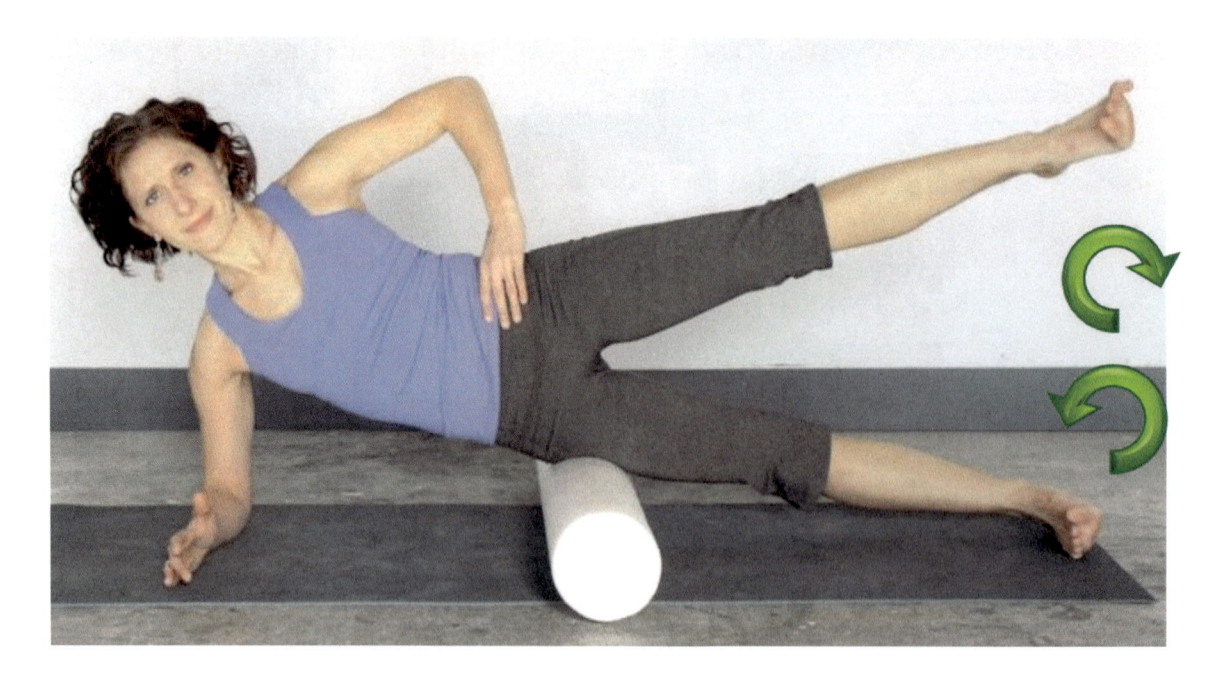

Circles: Phase 2 (circles forward & circles back)

Side Series:
Side Kicks: Bottom to Top

To Begin:
- Place the foam roller crosswise beneath the right hip, just below the bony protrusion.
- Stack the feet left on right, placing the right forearm on the floor running parallel with the foam roller.
- Lift the lower ribs to activate the lower obliques finding neutral from heels to crown.
- Draw the legs and feel parallel with each other, working not to lose neutral of the legs as well.
- INHALE, lift the top leg to hip height (this is not very high)
- Keeping the legs parallel, flex the upper foot and imagine you are hitting the ceiling with your outer most heel not the toes.
- EXHALE; lift the lower foot and leg to meet the floating top one, be careful not to sink into the lower ribs and obliques when lifting.
- INHALE; lower the leg to the floor.
- Repeat this movement 5 to 12 times.
- Repeat this series on the opposite side.
    - Variations:
        - *Pad the lower elbow if discomfort arises.*
        - *Practice this without the foam roller supporting the hip.*
        - *Try a mini ball under the bottom oblique.*
    - *2:1 Ratio*

Benefits:
- Here the hips are toned as with the other Side Series exercises.
- The adductors are toned to assist in lifting the lower leg.
- Be careful not to rock back when lifting the lower leg and over-use the hip flexors to lift.
- The inner thighs are an extension of the core and by working here we are strengthening the pelvic floor.

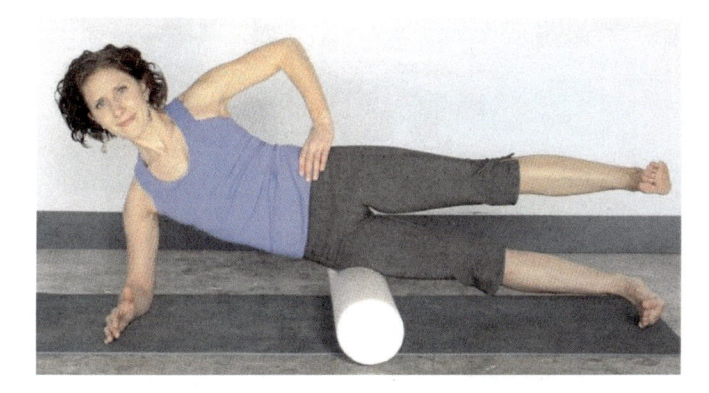

Bottom to Top Phase 1: Inhale

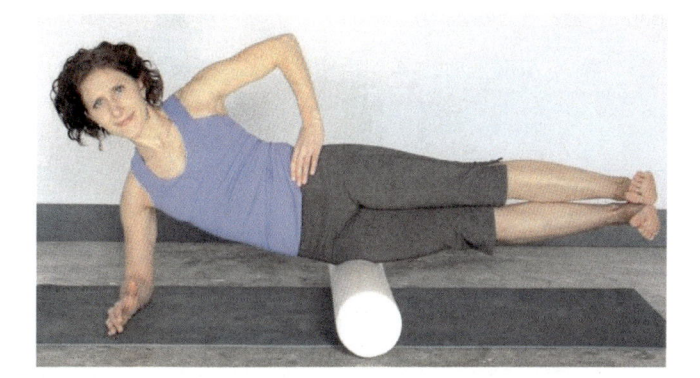

Bottom to Top Phase 2: Exhale

Side Series:
Oblique Lift:

To Begin:
- Place the foam roller crosswise on your mat.
- Come to your right hip and place the right forearm perpendicular with the foam roller.
- Press your forearm down towards the floor helping not to put all your bodyweight only on your elbow.
- Stack or stagger the feet with the knees slightly bent.
- Resting the top arm at its side open the front body completely.
- EXHALE, and lift the hips off the mat and allow the legs to lengthen fully.
- Remain lifted and confirm your core control.
- Hold this pose for 3 to 5 breaths.
- INHALE release back to the floor.
- Repeat the opposite side.
  - Variations:
    - Move as a series: EXHALE lift & INHALE lower (hover)
      - 3 to 5 times.
    - Modifications:
      - Omit the foam roller.
      - Place the top legs foot in front of the lower knee for more support.
  - 2:1 Ratio

Benefits:
- The obliques do a wonderful job of helping to support the spine on both sides.
- The obliques are a vital bridge between the pelvis and ribcage/shoulder girdle.
- Strength and stretch are important to help create the best balance in working the obliques not to create tightness at the attachments to the pelvis and rib cage.

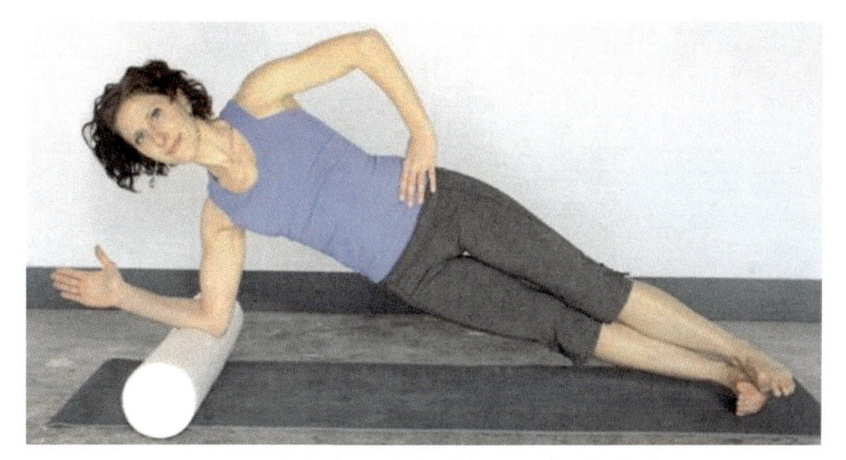

Oblique Lift Phase 1: Exhale

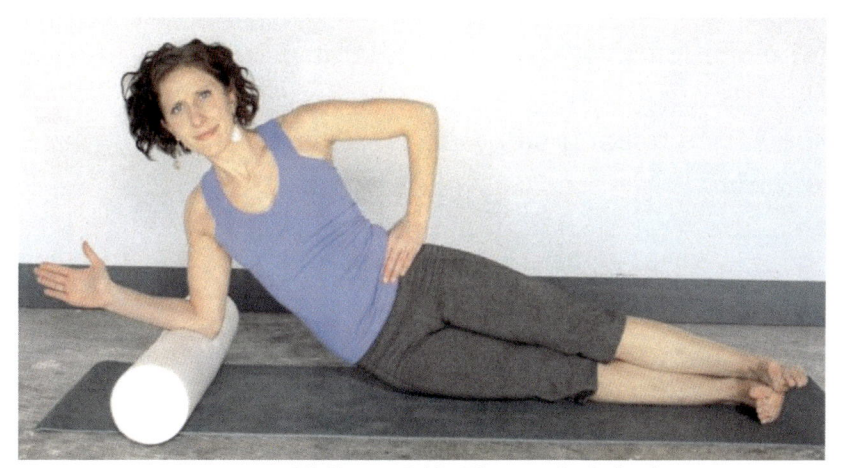

Oblique Lift Phase 2: Inhale

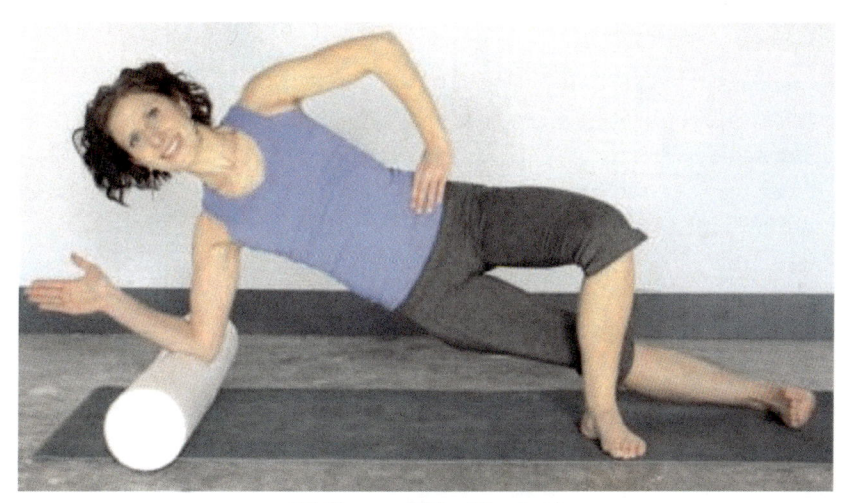

Oblique Lift: Variation

Side Series:
Mermaid Side Bend:

To Being:
- Place the foam roller at the right side of the mat crosswise with the mat.
- Stagger your legs off to the left, placing the right foot to touch the left thigh.
- Right hand rests on the roller, with the arm in an extended position.
- INHALE and lift the left arm palm up to shoulder height.
- EXHALE side bend to the right, rolling the foam roller away from the body and extending the left arm alongside the ear palm down.
- Keep both shoulders relaxed while side bending and the fold of the bottom elbow facing its fingers.
- INHALE; bring the body back upright and the left arm to shoulder height.
- Side bend to the left away from the foam roller, repeating the same process.
- Repeat this series to each side 3 to 5 times.
  - *Variations:*
    - *Use a small ball in place of a foam roller.*
    - *Omit the foam roller and perform the side bend, ensuring that you keep the shoulders relaxed.*
    - *Extend the top arm to the foam roller closing the torso to the floor and stretch.*
    - *Sit on a blanket if uncomfortable to sit on the floor to perform the movement.*
    - *Sit with both legs extended out in front (Staff Pose).*
  - *2:1 Ratio*

Benefits:
- This is a perfect movement of stretch and strengthen, or to practice after a side body strengthening series.
- Here, the lower back muscles are stretched, obliques worked and muscles of the shoulders are actively stretched and strengthened.

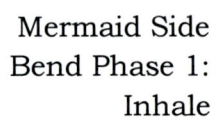

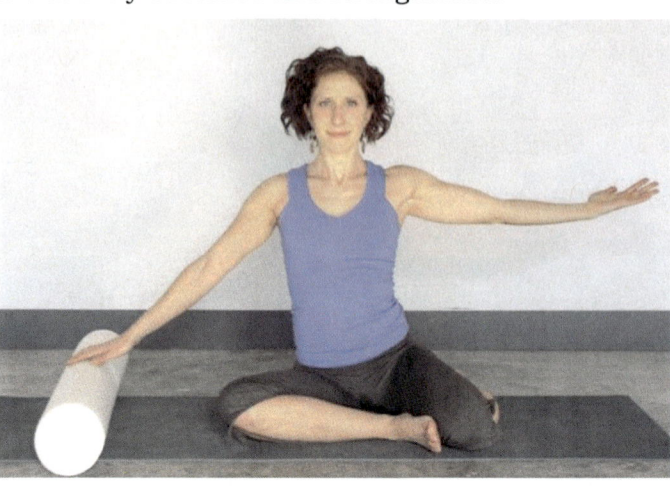

Mermaid Side Bend Phase 1: Inhale

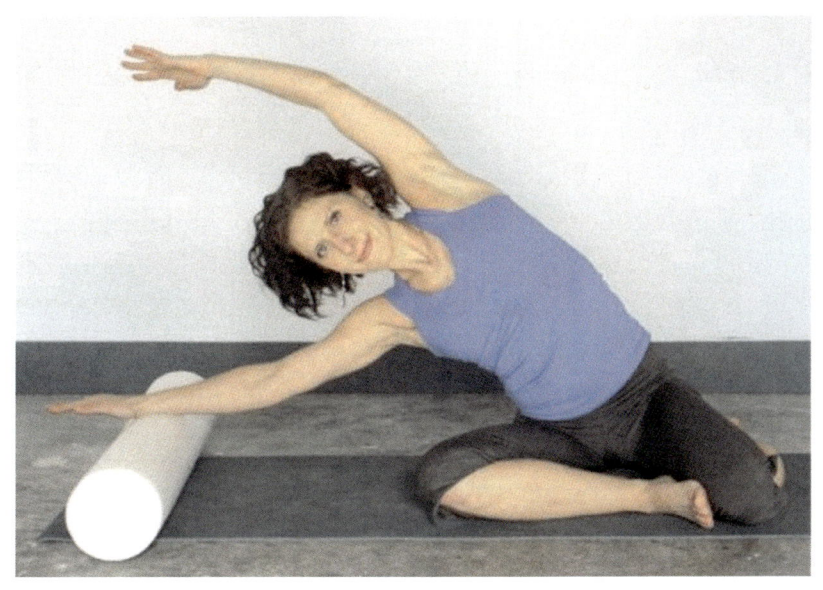

Mermaid Side Bend Phase 2: Exhale

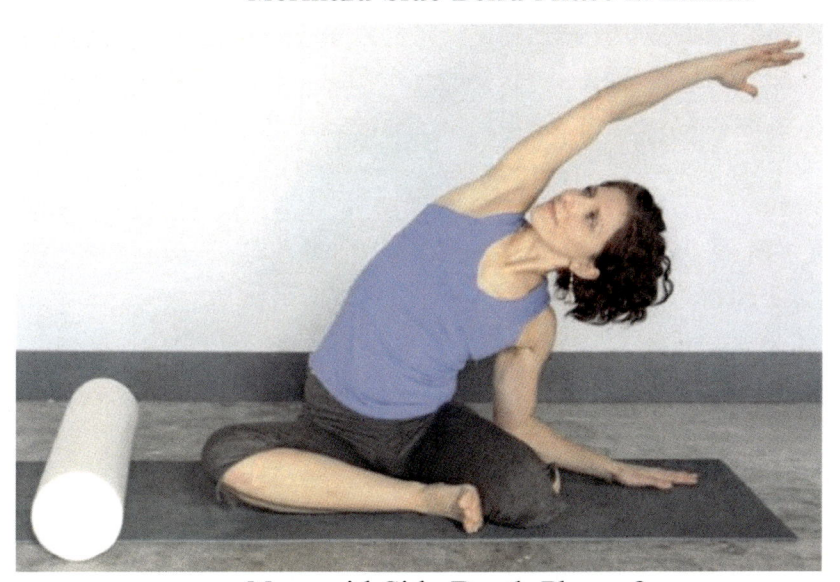

Mermaid Side Bend: Phase 3

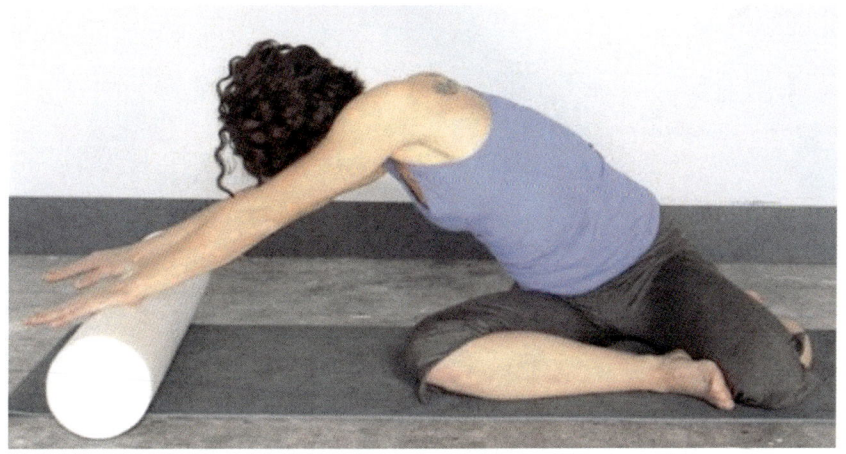

Mermaid Side Bend: Optional Extension

Side Series:
Side Push-Up:

To Being:
- Place the foam roller in front of the body parallel with your torso.
- Resting on your right hip, stack the legs and bend the knees.
- Place your left hand onto the center of the foam roller with the elbow aligning above or near the wrist.
- Cross your right hand to gently hold onto the left shoulder, hovering off the floor.
- EXHALE; lower the side body to hover at about roller level.
- INHALE and hold and hover.
- EXHALE, pressing into the foam roller keeping the side body strong return to center.
- Repeat this series 3 to 5 times, only performing the exercise as many times as you can effectively participate.
- Repeat this movement on the opposite side.
  - *Variations:*
    - *Try this without the foam roller, placing your palm on the mat.*
    - *Place your bottom hand to the rib cage if the chest is larger.*
  - *2:1 ratio*

Benefits:
- Here the deltoids, biceps, and triceps are all toned.
- The obliques are worked and muscles of the back are worked.
- Remember everything is an extension of the core so work from the inside out.

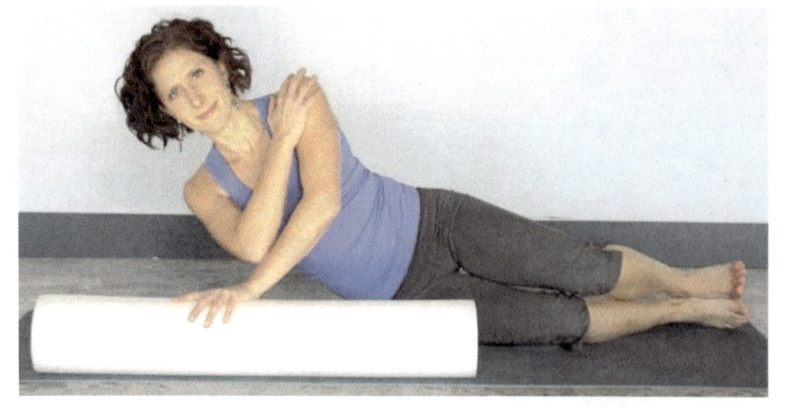

Side Push-Up Phase 1: Inhale

Side Push-Up Phase 2: Exhale

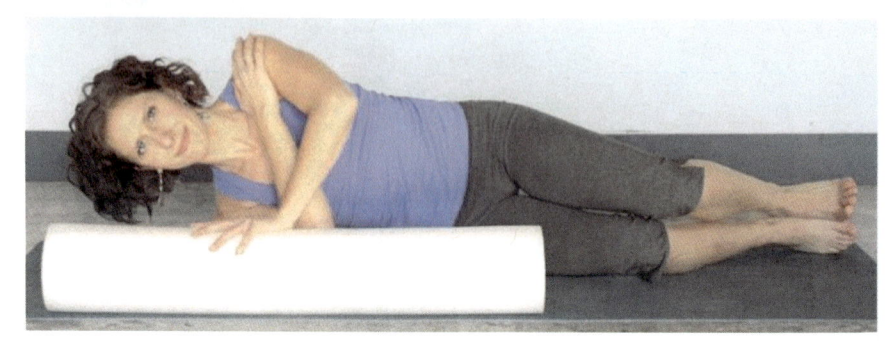

Rolling Lunge:

To Begin:
- Place the foam roller crosswise behind you, resting the top of the left foot on the foam roller.
- Check the front foot to be pointing forward.
- Find pelvic and spinal neutral and use the hands on the hip line to feel neutral.
- INHALE; begin to release your back leg to roll on the roller.
- Try not to let the body just roll back or forward, control the movement with the contraction of the legs and core, keep the torso up right.
- EXHALE, smoothly being to roll back to center, working to be steady and not to lean forward as you lift (imagine a book on your head).
- Repeat this movement 3 to 8 times.
- Repeat this on the opposite side.
  - *Variations:*
    - *Advanced:*
      - *Lift the arms as the body rolls back.*
      - *Add light hand weights (1-3 lbs.) held at the hips or used in the arm extension.*
  - *2:1 Ratio*

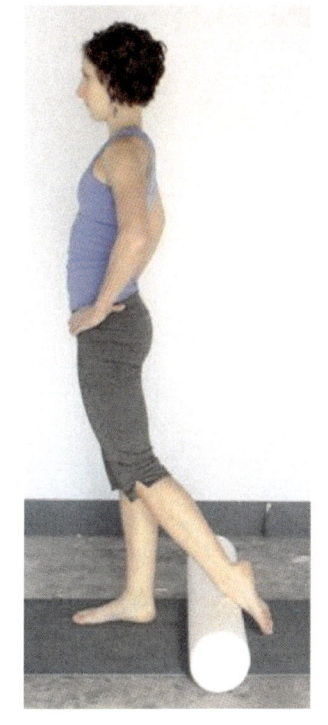

Rolling Lunge: Phase 1

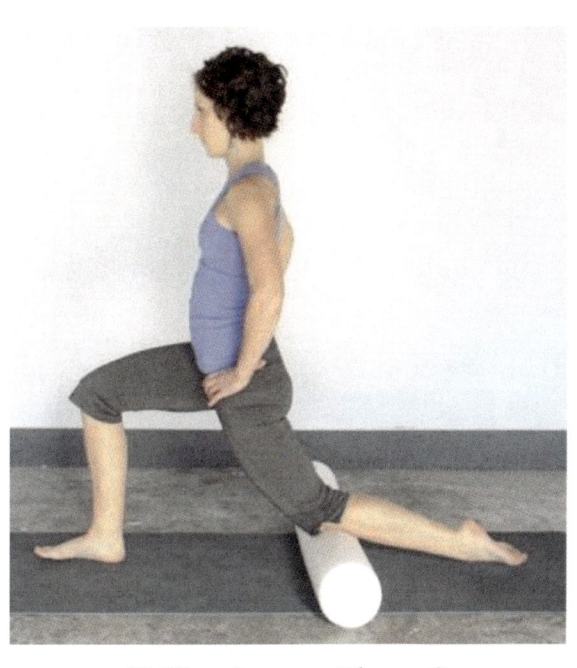

Rolling Lunge: Phase 2

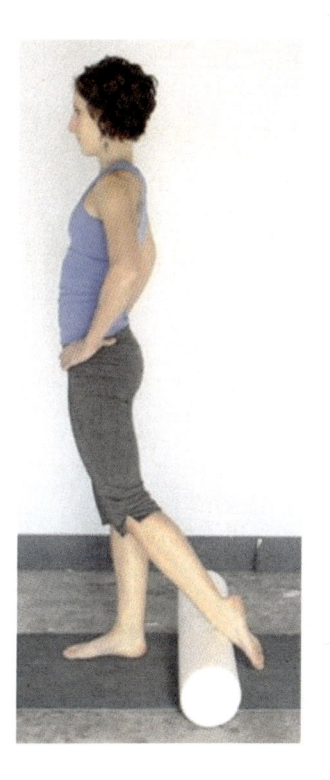

Rolling Lunge: Phase 3

Benefits:
- Rolling Lunge is a wonderful way to stretch the hip flexors, tone the legs and strengthen the glutes.
- Neutral is emphasized to assist in a more balanced posture.
- Adding the arm extension add a great lower back stretch and the latissimus dorsi is extended.
- When the glutes and hamstrings of the front leg are weak you will notice a lack of stability and the desire to lean to lift, think booty for a better backside.

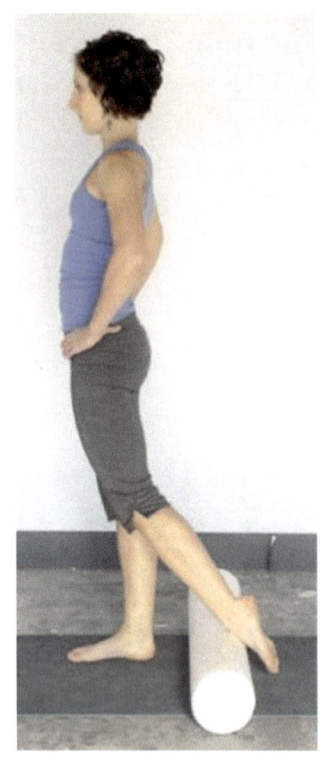

Advanced Rolling Lunge: Phase 1

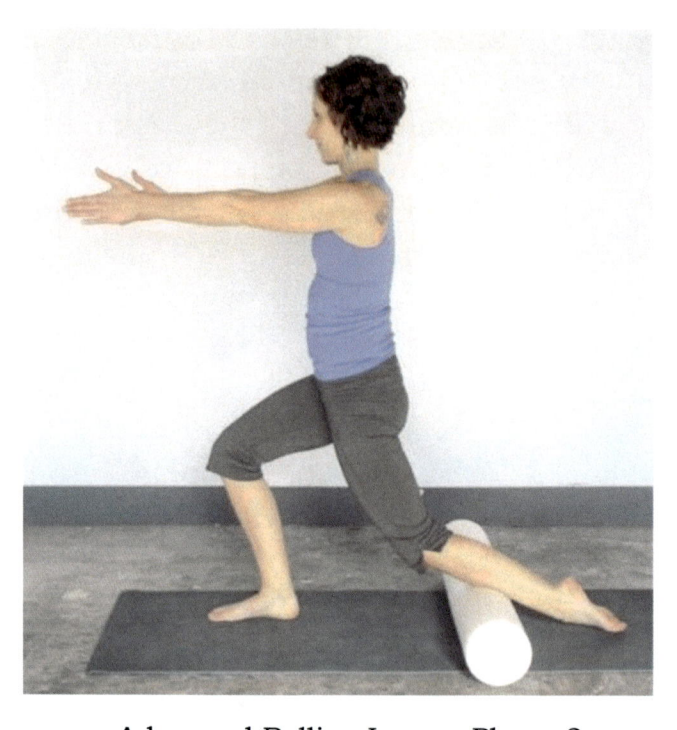

Advanced Rolling Lunge: Phase 2

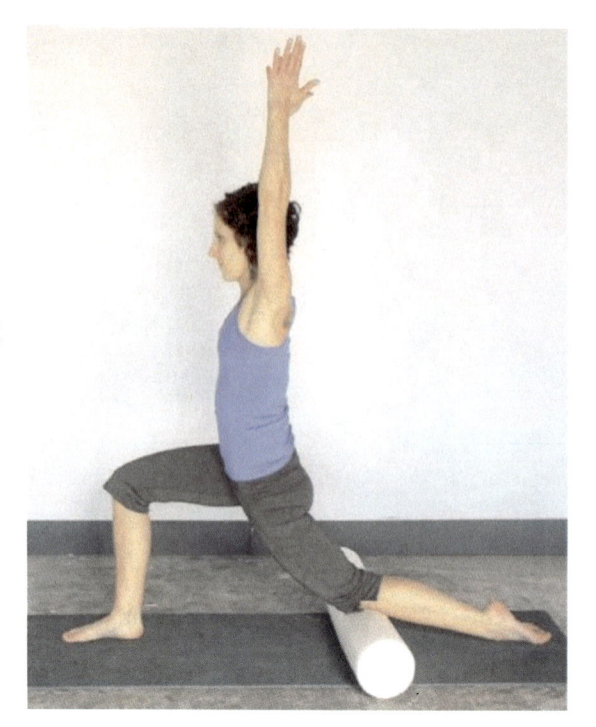

Advanced Rolling Lunge: Phase 3

Boat:

To Begin:

- Place the foam roller crosswise on the mat behind you.
- Sit onto the center of the foam roller.
- With the hands behind the foam roller, prop onto the finger tips and turn the hands to face away from the roller.
- INHALE; lengthen the entire spine, creating an open chest.
- EXHALE and lift the legs up to a table top position, drawing the ankle to knee level.
- Be mindful to keep the lower back long and the inner belly contracting to help release hip flexors.
- Remain here for 5 to 10 breaths working to stay steady.
- INHALE; slowly release the legs back to the floor.
    - Variations:
        - Advanced: Try extending the legs out to a 45° angle, keeping the legs parallel with each other, do not round the back.
        - Try this without the foam roller.

Benefits:

- Boat on the foam roller is a great core stability challenge.
- It offers the back body and the front body equal work and when aligned in neutral the body will use the proper muscles rather than ones that are already strong.
- If you notice the hip flexors straining chose a more modified version.

Boat: Version 1   Boat: Version 2

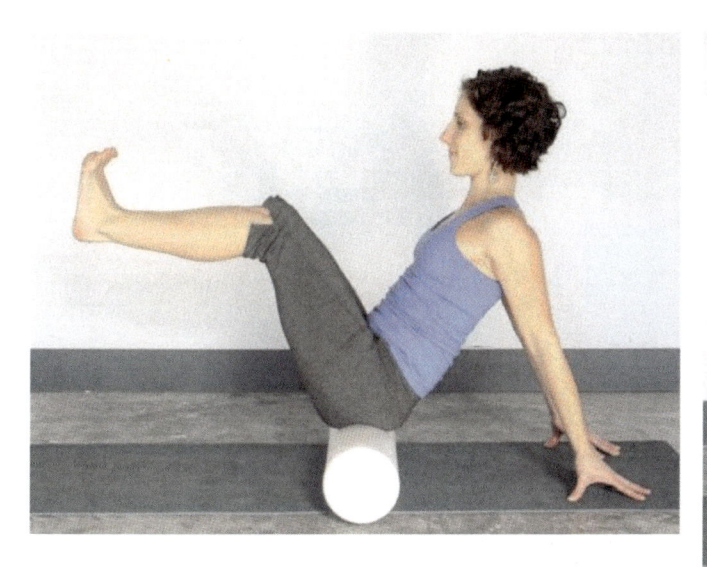

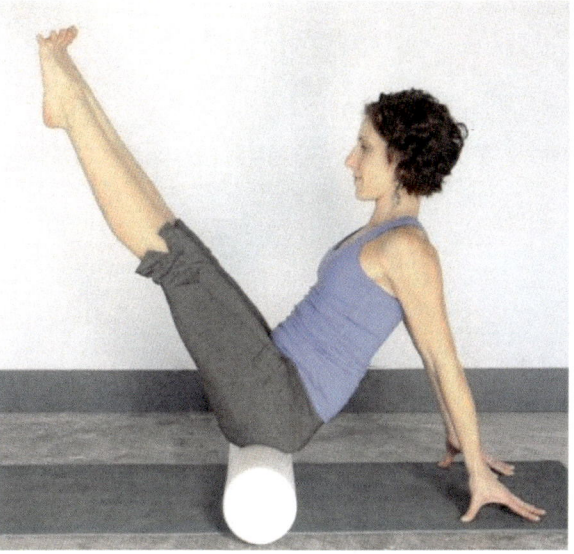

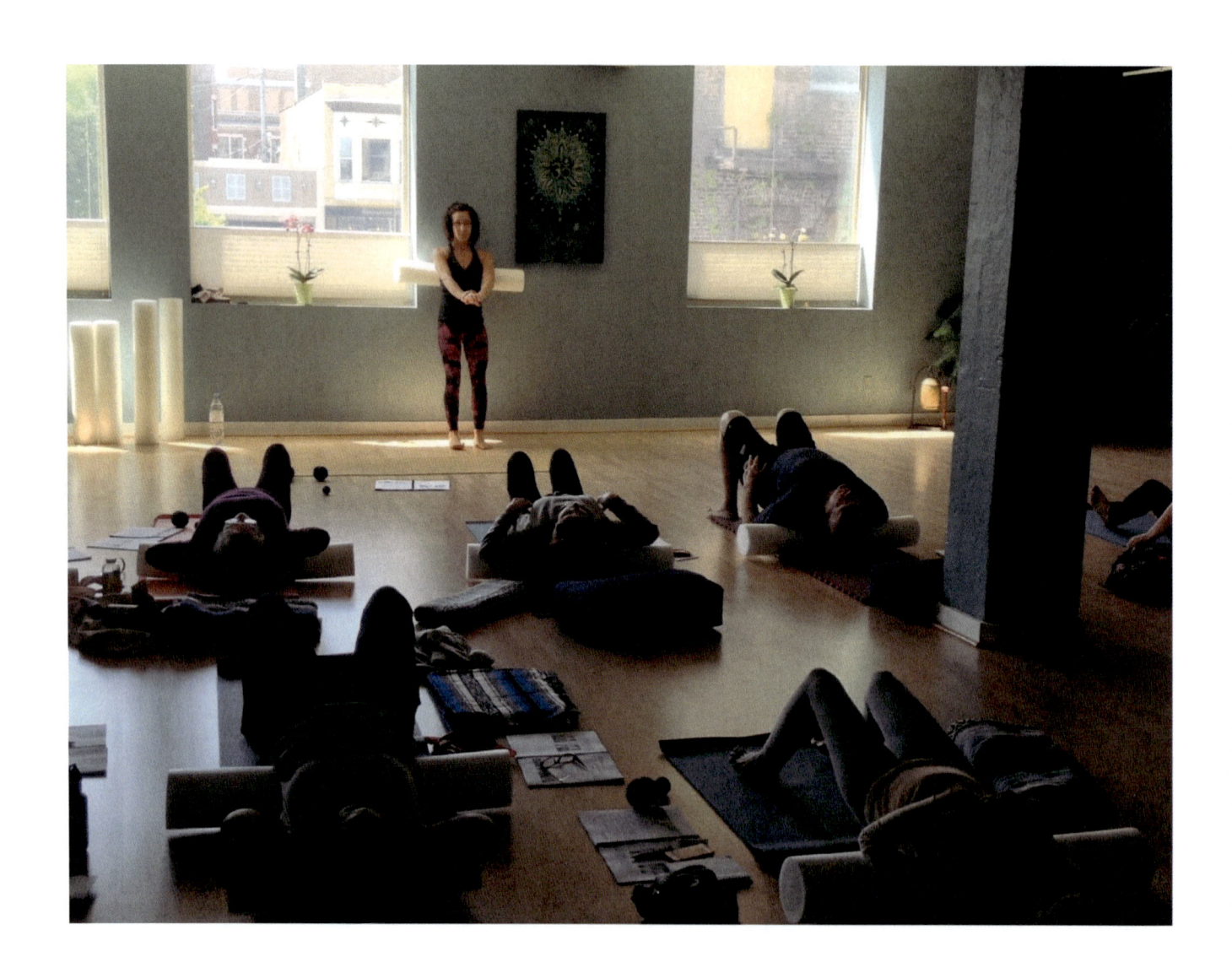

References:

Web Site Resources:

> ➢ Myers, Thomas: Blog, Courses
> https://www.anatomytrains.com/news/

Written Resources:

> ➢ Myers, Thomas: Anatomy Trains for Manual Therapists Workshop Guide
> ➢ Myers, Thomas: Anatomy Trains in Fascial Training Workshop Guide
> ➢ McGill, Stewart: Lower Back Disorders

Resources:

> ➢ **Dr. Cohen's Acuball**

http://www.acuball.com/

http://www.hopecorefitness.com/

> ➢ **Foam Rollers**

http://www.optp.com/

http://www.bpp2.com/physical_therapy_products/5250.html

http://www.hopecorefitness.com/

> ➢ **Fascial Research Congress**

http://www.fasciacongress.org/

Hope's Other Resources to compliment this workbook:

➢ Core Functional Fitness Functional Foundation Online Course
http://hopecorefitness.com/

➢ 5 Things you need to know about fascia
http://hopecorefitness.com/?p=858

➢ 3 Reasons why you should be foam rolling
http://hopecorefitness.com/?p=838

➢ Quick Core: Foam Roller Half Roll Up
http://hopecorefitness.com/?p=792

I want to personally thank you for your purchase of this workbook! This has been a constant job of updating and reworking in order to best serve my students. I am confident that no matter who you are, you will have found at least one, two, or maybe even ten moves in this workbook to better help your body, and if you are a fitness professional, to better help your students.

No matter what you do in life, remember that consistency and effort are two key components and for every slide down the mountain there is a way to climb back up. I wish each one of you well on your journey towards health, harmony and healing in everything that you do.

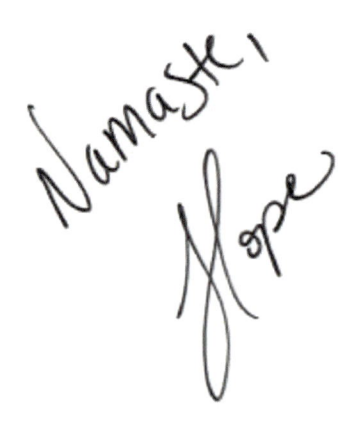

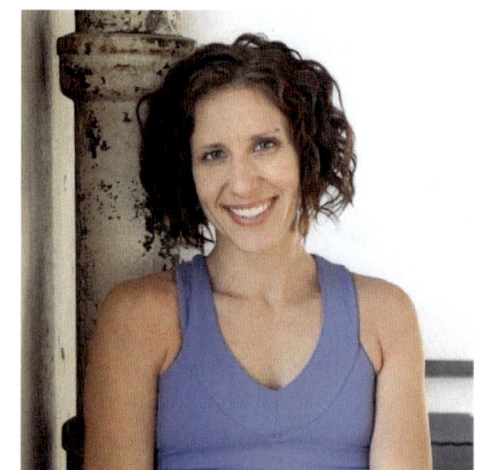

Namaste,
Hope

About the Author:

Hope Zvara is the creator of the HOPE Process: Helping Others Purposefully Excel. It is through this process that she helps willing individuals learn to live in their body's again using the three B's: Breathe, Body, Believe. With her off-the cuff perspective on life, Hope uniquely reworks both your mind and movement to ultimately transform you into the best damn version of yourself ever!

Hope is the creator of Core Functional Fitness by Hope Zvara®, director of HOPE Yoga Teacher Trainings and owner of Copper Tree Yoga Studio & Wellness Center in Hartford, Wisconsin. You can reach Hope directly at info@hopezvara or visit her s at www.hopezvara.com or www.hopecorefitness.com

Made in the USA
Monee, IL
20 September 2022